Love and Limits
In and Out of Child Care

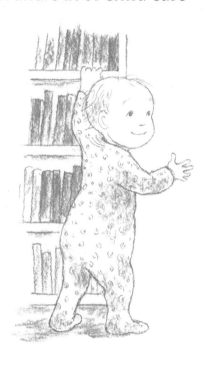

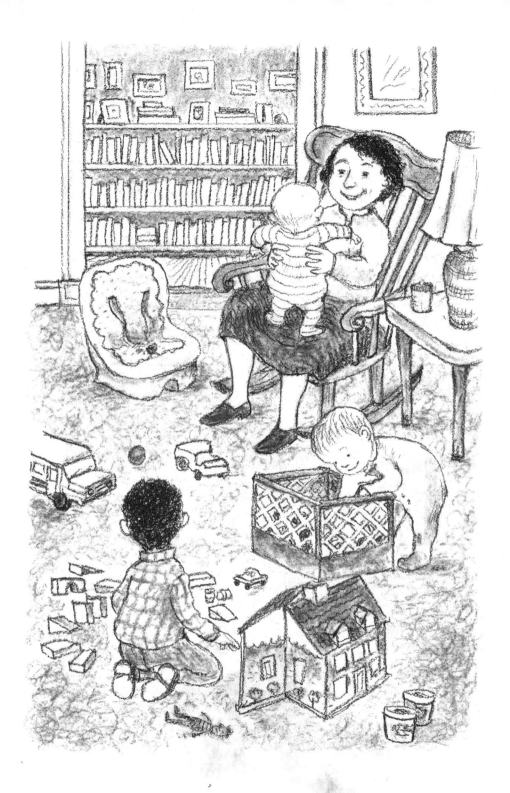

Love and Limits
In and Out of Child Care

What Your Child Care Provider and Your Pediatrician Want You to Know

Margaret Thomas

Richard Thomas

Lisa Dobberteen, M.D.

Illustrated by Susanna Natti

THE JOHNS HOPKINS UNIVERSITY PRESS | BALTIMORE

The Johns Hopkins University Press
2715 North Charles Street
Baltimore, Maryland 21218-4363
www.press.jhu.edu

Library of Congress Cataloging-in-Publication Data
Love and limits in and out of child care : what your child care provider
and your pediatrician want you to know / Margaret Thomas, Richard
Thomas, Lisa Dobberteen.
Thomas, Margaret, 1929–
      p.   cm.
   Includes bibliographical references and index.
   ISBN-13: 978-0-8018-8797-0 (hardcover : alk. paper)
   ISBN-13: 978-0-8018-8798-7 (pbk. : alk. paper)
   ISBN-10: 0-8018-8797-6 (hardcover : alk. paper)
   ISBN-10: 0-8018-8798-4 (pbk. : alk. paper)
   1. Child care. 2. Child rearing. 3. Child development. I. Thomas,
Richard, 1930 Mar. 9– II. Dobberteen, Lisa, 1956– III. Title.
   HQ772.T43 2007
   649'.1—dc22   2007031404

A catalog record for this book is available from the British Library.

Illustrations © Susanna Natti.

Special discounts are available for bulk purchases of this book. For more information,
please contact Special Sales at 410-516-6936 or specialsales

For our children, Wendy, Doug, Abby, and Andy,
and grandchildren, Teddy and Pru—
and all the children we have loved and cared for
throughout the years

CONTENTS

ACKNOWLEDGMENTS

Peggy is grateful for the support and friendship of the many parents who have entrusted their children to her care.

Lisa thanks her former teachers at Tufts–New England Medical Center Floating Hospital for Children and her current pediatric colleagues at the Cambridge Health Alliance who, every day, make the world a better place for children. Special thanks to David Link, M.D., and Jim Perrin, M.D., for their pediatric leadership and generosity of spirit as mentors and friends.

We are especially grateful for the guidance and support of Jacqueline Wehmueller, executive editor at the Johns Hopkins University Press. Jackie's wisdom, grace, and humor made this a better book in every way. We also thank other members of the Press staff, including Jennifer Gray and Juliana McCarthy, as well as our copy editor, Joseph Parsons.

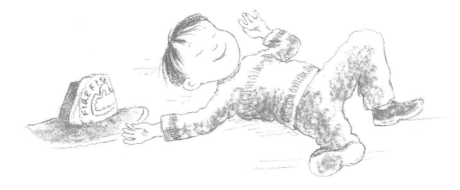

Lisa Dobberteen, M.D.

When my children were four years old and two and a half years old and I
was a busy pediatrician trying to juggle a part-time practice and still spend
time at home with my young children, I found myself in the midst of every
working mother's nightmare: no child care. I was anxious and frustrated.
Thanks to my training and clinical experience, I knew these years were
critical to healthy child development. I exhausted a string of unsuccessful
in-home caregivers.

There was the seemingly perfect, warm, older woman who complained
that my children were too active and quit after just two days. There had
been a lively, energetic young college student who was interested in early
child development; after helplessly crumbling in the midst of several of
my daughter's temper tantrums she quit, saying my daughter was too
difficult. A parent with her own child was unable to meet her child's needs
and care for my two children as well.

On and on. . . . In desperation, I searched frantically for other solutions.
I asked everyone I knew about his or her own child care options. The few
good places, either family child care or reputable centers, were all full and
had long waiting lists. I was at my wits' end. I even put a substantial de-
posit down at a for-profit center that came with all the warning signs: high
staff turnover, no windows, and the feel of a very dismal place to leave
children all day.

I'll never forget the day when a friend, our illustrator, Susanna Natti, said to my children's father, "I know a wonderful woman who cared for my children when they were young. I think she's still taking care of kids in her home. Why don't you give Peggy a call?"

That was the beginning of the best child care our family was privileged to enjoy and also the start of a wonderful friendship that has continued to thrive to this day. Peggy (Margaret Thomas, one of my co-authors) and I quickly discovered that we were kindred spirits, sharing a love of children, family, and a desire to make the world a better place. Over the years we have exchanged many stories and discussions of issues and controversies in child health, growth, and development. Those hours of talking, telling stories, laughter, and even shedding a tear or two have grown into this book.

We hope our expertise in our respective fields and our evident friendship makes this a useful, personal, and practical guide for new parents. Peggy has provided kind, nurturing child care in her home for more than forty-five years, and I have been a practicing pediatrician for more than twenty years. Each chapter begins with a narrative vignette drawn from Peggy's years of child care experience, followed by a discussion based on my professional expertise and review of the pertinent pediatric literature. (Note: The two narrative "voices" are in different colors so the reader can tell them apart.) We have changed the identifying characteristics of the children and families we've had the pleasure of encountering over these many years.

As a new parent, entering the world of young children can feel like traveling to a foreign country. We hope this will be a trusty guidebook to help you learn the language and, what's more, enjoy the trip as you move forward on your journey of parenting, the most rewarding journey in life.

Margaret Thomas

Writing this book with Lisa Dobberteen was great fun. The book's title evolved from our shared philosophy of what children need most: plenty of unconditional love from the caring adults around them and clear limits to help them understand, predict, and make sense of their world.

Limits are different from rules, but they can and should be used together. Limits are clear guidelines and boundaries set by adults for children that help them understand how to behave and how to stay safe in any setting. Rules are more formal and institutionalized, like the rules of a game or traffic regulations. We try to not shower children with a list of "no no's" but make our expectations clear as to how they should behave, and then give them abundant praise when they do behave.

Setting limits and modeling good manners for young children helps them develop a natural style of good behavior, which helps them feel at ease in any situation. Without exception, the children who leave my care have good manners and are sincere in expressing their love and respect for others. They are the sort of children both adults and other children welcome and enjoy.

Over the years, Dr. Dobberteen has often cared for children who attend my child care group. With affection they always call her "Dr. Lisa" and regard her as a friend and trusted grownup. The children often tell me about their visits for well-child checkups or for treatment when they are feeling sick. They never seem apprehensive, and that tells me a lot about Lisa, as children do seem to have a good sense of whom they can trust.

I believe Lisa and I both play important roles in the lives of the children we care for. I know that the parents of her patients consult her frequently on matters relating to behavior and development as well as medical issues. Similarly, the parents of the children I care for will sometimes consult me on weekends or evenings when something just doesn't seem right with their child. I may suggest parents call their pediatrician, or more frequently just reassure them if their child's behavior is a normal stage in development.

Over the years we have come to realize that the advice we each give is quite similar, and so this book was born. In caring for children Lisa and I stress love and believe you can't spoil a child with genuine affection. Children do need guidance from parents and caregivers, but we should never put a limit on giving hugs. We hope our book is useful in helping parents enjoy these wonderful and precious early childhood years.

Love and Limits
In and Out of Child Care

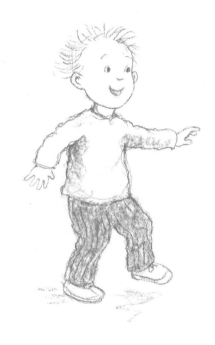

CHAPTER 1

A New Baby!

Becoming a Parent Today

Becoming a parent is one of life's major transitions. In two-parent families, couples will need to learn to share their intimate love for each other
with a totally dependent little stranger. Whether you are part of a couple
or a single parent, it's the total dependence of a helpless child on you that
can be so frightening.

When caring for a newborn, your old routine and daily schedule is
completely changed. The needs of the baby must come first. For most, it's
a joyful transition. Oh, you do lose some sleep for a while and may need
to adjust to staying home in the evening, but it doesn't matter. The baby
is a continuing delight.

With so many families in which both parents work, it's important
that both partners share in caring for the newborn. When the mother
is breastfeeding, she'll be the most sleep-deprived. The father or partner can pitch in by changing diapers, preparing meals, and cleaning the
house. Nowadays, most fathers are glad to accept these responsibilities—after all, they have been part of bringing up baby since that wonderful moment in the delivery room.

During the many years I have been providing child care, a new breed of
fathers has emerged. Every day these sensitive, caring fathers bring their
children to my home. I've also noticed that when couples are out for a
stroll, it's usually the father who is proudly pushing the baby carriage.

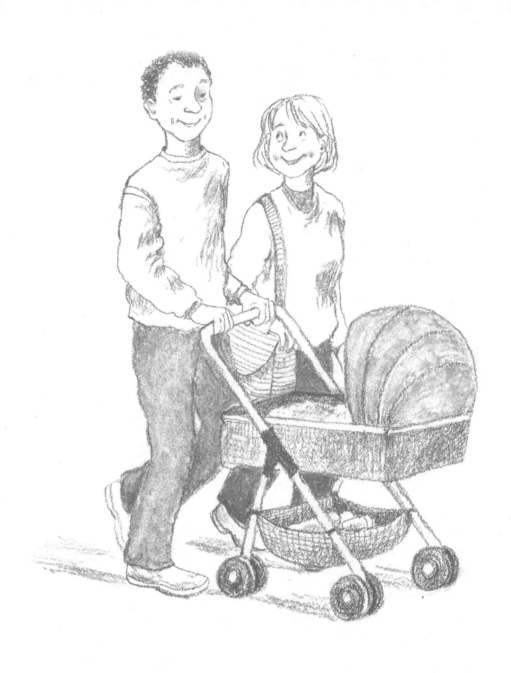

Things weren't always like this. These young dads are very different from the fathers most of the children of my generation grew up with. Where I lived as a child, the fathers were factory workers, transit drivers, garage mechanics, and cooks who spent their free time among men. Even during holiday family gatherings, they would cluster together near the refrigerator in the kitchen, while the women chatted together in the front room. Children, who were to be "seen and not heard," would go outside to play.

Many of these men seemed like heroes. During World War II, most had been away in the service. When they came home they seemed like mythical gods, to be feared and obeyed, yet revered for protecting us from harm. When children misbehaved, mothers would threaten, "If you're not good, I'll tell your father!"

It wasn't that the dads were mean, just that they were aloof figures and often not involved with their own small children. They might on occasion toss a ball outside with the boys, or on the weekend take us out for a drive and to get ice cream for a special treat, but in general they were removed from our lives.

During the war, most men not in the armed forces were doing work for the war effort: building ships, tanks, and bombers. Of course, some women had always worked outside the home to make ends meet, but it was during the war that legions of housewives entered the work force by working alongside the remaining men in the factories. For many women, working outside the home was a liberating experience. They were understandably disheartened after the war, when they were expected to return to a life of staying home and doing all the household chores.

Goodness, how times have changed. Most of the mothers of the children I take care of now are bright young women who are able to meet their career goals while successfully raising a family.

Fortunately, many employers now offer their staff flexible schedules, which are so helpful for working parents. Thanks to the computer and its connection to the Internet, many mothers and fathers are able to work part of the time at home.

Because few parents can afford a full-time, live-in nanny, they most often place their children in child care or nursery school. Many parents leave a young child with me for two or three days a week while they go to their offices and for the rest of the week work from home with a toddler playing at their side. The older children are in school most of the day, but their parents must juggle their work schedules to drive the children to soccer practice, music lessons, gymnastics, and numerous other after-school activities.

Mothers don't have to manage this busy schedule alone. Their husbands or their partners are an integral part of the family team. Before their children were born, fathers might have spent Saturdays mowing the lawn before settling down on the couch to watch a ball game. Now they do their share of the household chores and then play with their kids. When necessary, fathers will also take a personal or vacation day from work to care for a sick child.

In the past, parents could usually depend on someone in their large extended family to look after the children when they were at work. In some European countries this is still the case, although I'm told this is changing. My own sister lives in Rome, where most children, even after they marry, continue to live close by in their parents' neighborhood. With her daughter living across the street, my sister was available to care for her grandson, and to this day she continues to prepare all the family meals.

Although parenting today may be different from years ago, all new parents face the same fears: Will I be a good parent? Will I do the right thing,

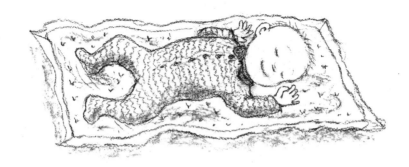

or say the right thing to my child? Will my child be healthy? Take heart in knowing that all good parents worry at least a little, and know you are doing your very best.

Peggy has described many of the issues parents of young children face today. All new parents have to come to terms with the overwhelming realization that their tiny baby is totally dependent on them. In the best of circumstances, when a child is wanted and planned for at the right time, that realization evolves naturally, as part of the parents' own developmental progression.

After you bring that tiny baby home, the first few weeks fly by in a sleep-deprived blur. Parents are (understandably) consumed by the all-important matters of feeding the baby and getting some sleep. Gradually, as the feeding and sleep issues are worked out together by parents and the baby, most parents gain a confident sense of their identity as parents.

I notice this in my office, when I compare families and their babies at visits during the first month and the visit when the baby is two months old. By two months the baby is usually sleeping better, feeding is well established, and, most important, the parents know their child.

I am always delighted by the transformation. Those sleepy, confused, and uncertain parents who came when their baby was just a few days and then a few weeks old become confident, warm parents who handle their two-month-old baby with ease. "That's a hunger cry," the dad will announce, and hand his daughter to the mom to feed. "He needs his diaper changed," the mom will say, and efficiently and cheerfully take care of what makes a nonparent gasp.

With two-parent families, a significant transformation occurs in the context of the adults' relationship. Even the strongest of couples has to readjust when they become a family of three. No longer do the needs of two adults come first; now the needs of the baby take precedence over all.

It is helpful for parents to address their relationship directly and often and to get in the habit of attending to it early on in their career as parents. Take up all those offers from friends and family who are eager to sit for the baby.

As the baby settles in, get in the habit of deliberately setting aside some adult time, as preventative maintenance for your relationship.

A word about the relationship between breastfeeding mothers, their husbands or partners, and infants is in order here as we think about the transformation that occurs as adults become parents. The dyad of a breastfeeding mother and her infant is incredibly intense and all encompassing. It is understandable when the father or other parent feels left out.

Fathers or other parents may often feel, too, that there is nothing they can do when their baby cries except hand the infant back to the mother to nurse. The most helpful way to move beyond these feelings is to realize that what you do to support the breastfeeding mother of your child is equally important and meaningful.

You will work out your own ways of soothing your crying baby, such as rocking, singing, or other comforting measures. You will marvel at the healthy growth of your baby, fed by her mother, and you will marvel at what her mother, your wife or partner, is able to do. And in supporting her—by changing the baby, cooking for both of you, keeping the house picked up—you will find your relationship becomes deeper and stronger.

Children grow and change fast, and sometimes parents are wistful about what is left behind. However, as children grow, the best parents cheer them on. I love to see parents who delight in each milestone, look forward to what their child will do next, and remember fondly what they used to do.

Parents of two-year-olds who have a second child will say, "He seems so grownup to me now, compared to the baby!" Parenting today occurs against a backdrop of our lives busy with jobs, family, and community activities, so it is essential to live in the present, enjoy each stage with your child, and realize that childhood will move quickly.

Another stage in the process of becoming a parent today is the decision to have a second child or subsequent child. Families pursuing adoption go through this stage as well. Is your family complete with one child or are siblings in your child's future?

Many parents with more than one child have told me over the years that all through the infancy and toddler years of their first, they still felt like they were learning and practicing. Only after the arrival of their second child, with the ease that comes from the realization that, yes, they do know what they're doing, did they truly feel complete in their transformation as parents.

Another transformation that occurs in families is when the grandparents realize that their children are now parents. This is particularly and understandably difficult for teen parents, whose own parents probably feel they have some parenting left to do. Even when the new parents are mature adults, however, some grandparents interfere. They are certainly well meaning, but they must step back and let the new parents succeed in their new roles. In the best of circumstances grandparents should support their children, help when asked, and enjoy their grandchildren.

As your children grow, you will find each transition is also significant for you as a parent. The first day of kindergarten is one such moment, even if your child has been in child care or preschool. Elementary school is different. Enjoy those milestones for your child—and for you as a parent.

Milestones in parenting evolve as your children grow. This became all too clear to me as I took that leap of faith and helped my teenagers learn to drive. Seeing them go off to college is another, and down the road, graduate school or starting a career, marriage, and children in some order or another.

Enjoy the moments and the milestones. Remember that you are becoming an expert in parenting your child, and he or she is becoming an expert in being your child. Take lots of pictures, write everything down, and live in the present. You will be glad that you did.

CHAPTER 2

Love and Limits

Raising Happy, Secure Children

Parents often ask me how I care for several children throughout the day and remain so at ease. Based on their own experiences with their children at home, parents assume that my day must be equally hectic. It really isn't.

The children are rarely noisy, and if it's "play noise" such as laughing or talking together, of course, I don't mind. I do not allow screaming, climbing on furniture, or running in the house. It's a matter of common sense, because someone might get hurt. Crazy, erratic, and wild behavior disturbs the other children as well as me. It's important to set limits for a child. If you are clear and consistent about what is allowed and what is not permitted, children will understand. It's really just teaching good manners.

Discipline isn't a popular word these days, although it seems to be making a comeback. *Positive reinforcement of rules* may be a better term. When it is necessary to correct a child, I always make direct eye contact, which assures full attention. When I say "No!" in a strong voice, the child usually obeys. On the rare occasion when I have to give a "time out" and send the child to "the corner," it's only for a brief time. For a preschool child a minute can seem like an eternity.

Children are wonderfully observant, and they rise to the expectations of the adults and environment around them. They appreciate and respond to routine. I experienced this during my own childhood, when my mother died when I was five years old. In my large family, we had to learn to take care of each other and ourselves. With my father and older siblings off at work, we younger children were what were referred to as "latchkey kids." Limits and assigned tasks after school kept us busy and together as a motherless brood. During World War II, I was sent to St. Vincent de Paul, a Catholic boarding school, and I loved the fact that the sisters supervised the children closely every hour of the day. We always knew exactly what was expected of us, and I felt secure. It is a lesson I've always remembered.

Setting clear limits helps children make sense of their world and predict what comes next.

The daily activities in my day care group follow a routine: morning play, lunch, naps after lunch, a story hour, followed by more play or a children's video, if allowed by parents. *The Mouse and the Motorcycle* and *Charlotte's Web* are charming video adaptations of beloved children's stories. The day has a very pleasant feel to it, and the children can always anticipate what comes next.

Over the years, I've cared for children who completely dominate life at home by making unreasonable demands yet are perfectly cooperative during the day with me. It's understandable that busy parents are reluctant or ambivalent about disciplining their children during their few hours together. They want their time together to be happy, "quality" time. But again, children need limits. A successful family is a shared enterprise and a happy partnership between the adults and children with the parents always firmly in control.

Children respond to reasonable expectations. I once cared for a child who was with us from the age of two months to three years old, when he went off to preschool. His parents had a big problem: the child would get up early in the morning, sneak out of the house, cross the street and wander about the neighborhood. It was a very dangerous game.

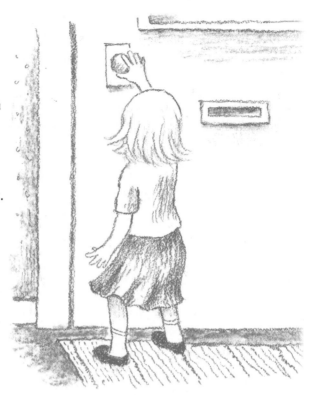

I keep the doors in our house locked, as we live on a busy street. The older children can reach the deadbolt and doorknob but are instructed not to open the door at any time without permission. The little boy known for wandering at home never opened the door at my house, as he knew exactly what was expected of him at my house, and exactly what the limits were. I will ask a child who is old enough to reach the lock to open the door in the evening for Mommy or Daddy at pick-up time. They love to do it, as they feel grown up enough to help me, and understand the special nature of an earned privilege.

I find it surprising that professional parents, who understand the importance of clear guidelines and reasonable expectations in the workplace, are reluctant to set up the same structure in their homes. It's as if they just don't expect their children to behave. It's a pity, as it is just so much harder later for a child to adjust to the limits expected in preschool and beyond.

The safety of the children in my care is a paramount concern at all times. Toys and behavior have to be safe. We have several kinds of building blocks, a doll house with family figurines, stuffed animals, and a favorite yellow school bus, all playthings which have been carefully chosen over the years to be fun and safe, and which inspire imaginative play. Children can bring a favorite toy to my house as long as they are willing to share with the others, and as long as it is a safe toy. You know how often children put things in their mouths, especially during teething. That's why I ask parents not to bring small items such as marbles, coins, or anything with sharp edges.

Sharp edges! Now, here's an example of a parent who was unable to refuse a two-and-a-half-year-old's unreasonable demand. One morning little Nancy came in carrying a small plastic bag. When I asked her mother what she had in the bag, she calmly replied that it was a box cutter, including the blade.

Her mother went on to explain that she wanted to keep the box cutter with her to remind her of her daddy. "I tried to take it away, but Nancy wouldn't give it to me." Now remember, Nancy was only two and a half, and she couldn't take the box cutter away from her? Why was she allowed to have it in the first place? Wouldn't you expect an intelligent adult to be able to keep a dangerous item out of a young child's reach?

I simply asked Nancy to "give the bag to Peggy," and she handed it to me without a fuss. We left the box cutter in its plastic bag on top of the bookcase for the day, out of reach of all the children. Needless to say, I told her mother that a box cutter had no place in our playgroup, and to please never bring anything like that again.

It is not unkind to set limits. In fact, you are doing your children a disservice if you are not teaching them to be cooperative, polite, and considerate. I've cared for several children over the years who were gifted and surely destined for many academic honors. Those are special gifts to be treasured, but a child needs more than intelligence to get along in this world successfully. Parents should stress that it is important to get along with and work well with others; to share, to be kind to others, and to obey their parents. It may seem old fashioned, but saying "Please" and "Thank you" can take you a long way in life.

Don't we all quake inside at the thought of Peggy's story of the little girl with the box cutter, and yet worry that some time we also as parents have given up too easily with our own children and yielded on a matter that just wasn't right? As in all matters of raising healthy young children, the best techniques in encouraging good behavior and setting limits are often those that take the most time and effort on the parent's part. Setting limits and being clear start at an early age. For most children and parents this becomes an issue when babies start to be mobile, and certainly is an issue for all toddlers striving for independence in the eighteen months to three- year-old period.

Pick your battles. You don't need to make the house full of rules and "No!" but you do need to set clear limits about issues of safety from an early age. A newly crawling baby or early walker can learn and understand "No" when approaching the stove. That is something they just can't touch. Similarly, a child old enough to walk can learn that she always holds an adult's hand when crossing the street. No holding hands? Then no crossing the street to the fun location you were planning to enjoy together.

The key to setting limits successfully is consistency. "No" has to always mean "No" and not "maybe" or it will lose its effectiveness. A child who

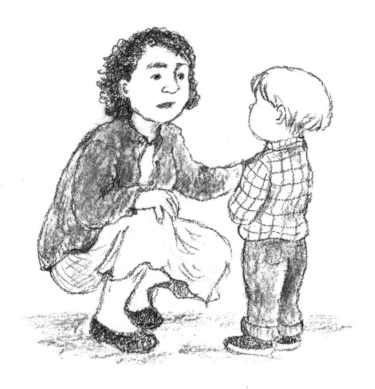

is refusing to hold hands may be testing, and you as a parent have to pass that test with flying colors. That is a perfect time to sit down on a nearby step and say, "Well, if you can't be safe and hold hands crossing the street, we'll just have to sit here until you're ready." And then, just wait. A child who tries to bolt should be told "no" firmly, and gently restrained if necessary in a big hug. Sometimes there is no stronger will than a toddler's, and if she won't change her mind, you may have to turn around and go home. Children are very observant, so be certain that the next time, that little hand finds its way into yours to cross the street.

Setting limits also requires some flexibility to change plans if need be as a parent to reinforce a concept. This is very difficult in our busy lives, when an errand such as a trip to the grocery store feels like it has to be squeezed in on the way home from day care. Terminating a shopping trip when a child is having a temper tantrum stirs up dark thoughts of "When am I ever going to get the shopping done?" but is essential if you want to demonstrate that "If you can't calm down now, we'll have to go right home."

Sometimes there are creative ways to shift household tasks to other times during the week or even take up a friend's offer to pick up a few things. Many parents trade off household tasks and try to be flexible; late nights are great times to zip through the near-empty grocery store on your own as opposed to trying to complete a necessary task with a tired toddler in tow. The years with young children are also times in your life to let go of the drive for perfection. Your children won't remember any gourmet meals the family shared when they were little, but they will grow up with a fond sense of fun times spent together playing with their parents.

"Time-out," as Peggy has nicely described in the family day care setting, is an excellent technique to emphasize to a child that they have done something that is not acceptable. The child needs to be somewhere—in a chair, on the step, in their room, even in their crib if they are an active toddler who can't sit still, for a brief time. This accomplishes many things: it is not fun, the child learns you mean business, and it takes the child away from you, and your positive attention, which they crave most of all. A good rule of thumb is one minute per year of age, so a two year old gets a two-minute time-out.

For recalcitrant children you may need to get an old-fashioned kitchen timer that rings when the time is up. If the child leaves the time out space ahead of schedule show them you are setting the timer again, then insist she go back until the bell rings. Again, stick to the program. I find when parents tell me "Time-out doesn't work" it is because they have been worn out by a strong willed two year old, and haven't been able to follow through consistently. This is very much in your child's best interests, so persevere. When the time-out is over, no more admonishments. Just be pleasant and move on.

Try, whenever possible, to "catch your child" being good. Positive reinforcement for desired behaviors is always much more effective than playing catch up trying to get rid of negative behaviors. Your child adores you, and you are their most powerful role model, so always be sure to model the behaviors you would like to inspire in your children. Careful use of language, using please and thank you, thanking others around you, and using warm nurturing tones all help your child to see how to behave, and how to treat others.

Physical punishment, such as spanking with the hand or beating with an object, has absolutely no place in caring for children. Even if you were spanked as a child, that does not mean that spanking has any place in raising your own children. Too often children are spanked in the heat of the moment. It teaches them that grownups can hurt children, and that violence is an answer to a problem, neither of which are helpful lessons for growing up as a kind, nurturing adult. Even the littlest child can learn the meaning of "no," and you will feel immensely better knowing you have encouraged your child with positive loving discipline and limits.

Parents need to be each other's best allies in setting limits. Children have an uncanny ability to sniff out disagreements, and even a toddler will pick up on one parent saying yes and the other saying no. Try to save your discussions about how to discipline your children for when the children are asleep, then give each partner a chance to speak. Each parent grew up in a family (or even different cultures) with very different styles of parenting, and it may take a number of discussions to reach your own new agreement about how you as a family will raise your children.

A word about discipline and single parenting is appropriate here. Families come in all sizes and configurations, and many times an adult is parenting one or more children on their own. The lack of another partner can be frustrating and exhausting, and discipline on your own can feel overwhelming. Once again, try to be consistent, as those limits are all up to you to set and reinforce.

A single parent may not have the luxury of trading off time for household chores or even relaxation, so be creative. If you always have to shop with your children, make it an activity. Shop early in the day when the store is quiet and the children are at their best. Let them each pick out a new fruit or vegetable to try later, and make up alphabet games about what is in each row. Children love rituals and routine, so a simple stop for an ice cream cone or trip to the park on the way home from the store that they can look forward to is a big incentive.

We all know, as adults, that we don't always get what we want. Life is full of setbacks of all sizes, and learning to cope with them creatively and not being overwhelmed is a very important life task. Setting limits and helping your child cope provide an important beginning to growing up to be a flexible, creative adult who is capable of handling challenges and overcoming frustration. Teaching your children to be kind, polite, and considerate of others is rewarding for you as a parent, and equips them with the skills that are essential in today's complex world.

CHAPTER 3

The Nuts and Bolts of Child Care

Hours, Logistics, and Communicating with Your Caregiver

Most of the children in my care are referred to me by word of mouth. When expectant mothers and new dads start looking for a child care placement they usually begin by asking friends and acquaintances in the community, "Who took care of your baby when you went back to work?" Sometimes it is entirely by chance that new families hear of me. Someone knows a friend of a friend whose child stayed with Peggy, and they suggest giving me a call. When they telephone, I ask parents to come by my house for a visit during the day, if at all possible, so they can observe the children at play. It is essential that we take the time to interview each other. We *both* have to be sure that my home will be a comfortable fit for their child.

During our interview, I discuss my schedule to be sure that it fits the family's needs. Normally I'm available to care for children between eight a.m. and six p.m., Monday through Friday, although I can be flexible because parents occasionally do have early appointments. These days most of the children are with me part time during the week, usually arriving in the late morning or at noon after attending a preschool.

Both of our children are married and have settled in England, and we like to plan a month-long visit there in mid-July each year. I don't ask for a paid vacation, so I feel comfortable in setting my dates when it works best for my own family. It has never been a problem, and parents plan ahead for alternative child care during that time. Many families plan their own vacations during the time I'm away, so the children and I excitedly go off on our adventures at the same time!

During the rest of the year, I expect to be paid for the number of hours each family schedules for their child even when the child misses time because of family travel or illness. I also emphasize to parents that, out of fairness to the other children and their own child, sick children should stay home. This means if the child has a fever or is too uncomfortable to participate in our daily activities, she should stay home for more rest and quiet. This can be challenging for parents, especially if they take the child's temperature in the morning and find it normal but later in the day, while with me, the fever creeps back up. The best time to take a child's temperature is around four in the afternoon the day *before* you make a decision about keeping the child at home.

In our initial interview the parents and I also discuss lunch, which I provide, nap time for older children, and infant feeding. We talk about play, the stories I read, and my philosophy of raising children with clear limits and lots of love. Because I believe it is important for parents to know me well before they leave their children in my care, I describe my family life. I also encourage parents to ask questions, and frankly I'm disappointed if they don't ask many! Parents need to ask me lots of questions to help them decide whether I am the right caregiver for their child.

Years ago I knew a former schoolteacher who cared for children. She had the opposite philosophy and didn't share information with the families of the children she cared for. She would meet the parents at the door and never even allowed them to enter her home. I thought this very odd at the time and still do.

Parents should know everything about their day care provider and the atmosphere in which their children are cared for.

Often after our talk, parents ask to reserve a place at once. Because it is such an important decision, I always ask them to think it over carefully for a day or so and then call me back. I give preference for open slots to parents who return with their second, third, or even fourth child. I consider it a true compliment that mothers have even been known to plan their pregnancies according to when I'll have an opening available. "Going to Peggy's" becomes a family tradition, and I enjoy keeping in touch with the older children who have "outgrown" me while I care for their younger siblings.

When parents leave in the morning, the children and I wave at the window. In the evening when each child leaves I ask for a hug and wave to them at the window. Sometimes a child will ask to come by to see me on a Saturday, just to visit. Halloween is a wonderful time with visits from all the children from my group, both present and former members, all dressed up in their costumes. It's a tradition, which they continue even into high school age, and I love seeing them all.

Many of the parents of children in my care have come to our annual Christmas party for years. They call me around Thanksgiving to ask when I'll be having the party. It's always a fun time, when I serve the Italian specialties that are part of my own family's traditions. Friends of all faiths gather around our piano to sing "Jingle Bells" and share in the glow of a happy time.

Peggy has outlined the important essentials in communicating with your caregiver and how to establish a good relationship from the beginning.

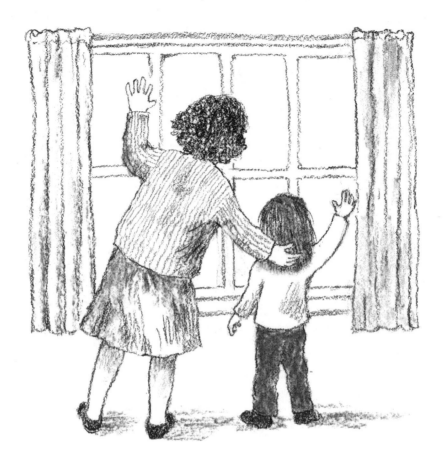

I couldn't agree more. In fact, along with her wonderful loving ways with children, one of the things that impressed me most during my "interview" with Peggy was her businesslike approach to running a family child care center in her home.

As I mentioned earlier, I had experienced many ups and downs with a variety of child care providers and options and was at my wit's end to find a good situation for my two young children. Hearing Peggy, in a straightforward fashion, outline the day and her expectations of me was such a relief and was very appealing. "This," I thought, "is a woman who will not let me down!" I was right, but little did I know what a rich relationship was beginning for my whole family that continues to this day.

Choosing the right type of child care is an individual decision. It depends on your family's needs, financial factors, and what options are available in your community. Large child care centers offer extended hours and relative stability and may be open some holidays and weekends. Smaller, not-for-profit child care centers operated by faith organizations or community groups may offer more informal care in a fashion closely aligned with your family's values. Family child care offers a homelike setting, one or two caregivers, and a small number of children for your child to interact with. A nanny or babysitter who cares for your child in the home offers the most consistency and convenience but is certainly the most expensive. For families fortunate to have a relative willing to provide child care, rejoice; still, to make sure the arrangement works smoothly, be sure to agree on all the details in a businesslike fashion just as you would with a non-family member.

Regardless of the setting, the important questions are the same in choosing the right child care for your child. Pay very close attention to how you feel when meeting the family child care provider or the staff at a center. Do they truly love children? Can you happily go off to work each day and leave your child in their care? The quality and experience of the caregivers are paramount, so getting information about the staff, their training, and their length of time at that particular center or family child care is crucial. A center with high turnover, a family child care that starts and stops with interruptions, or nannies that quit with no warning will all be distressing for both you and your child.

Each state has regulatory agencies, such as the Office for Children in Massachusetts, which oversee the care of children; reviewing what is required in your state is useful before starting to look for child care. Many are based in each state's department of public health or department of education. A good place to start is your state's Web site. The National Association for the Education of Young Children (NAEYC) is a wonderful advocacy and educational organization with a helpful Web site. The organization sets standards for preschools and larger child care facilities and provides a variety of resources and training for professionals and parents.

When making sure that the caregiver and setting is right for you and your child, safety and health issues need to be considered:

» Is the home or center free of sharp edges?
» Are hazardous equipment, chemicals, and cleaning supplies locked up?
» Is the telephone number of the local Poison Control Center readily available?
» Are all electrical plugs covered?
» Does the provider or staff know basic first aid and CPR?
» Are all children immunized in accordance with the regulations mandated by your state's Department of Public Health?
» What is the plan in the event that one child becomes ill at the child care home or center, and how will you and the staff or provider handle that situation together?

The question of how to handle sick children is complex. Certainly if you have a caregiver who comes to your home and your child is sick, in most cases that person can continue to care for your child. As Peggy so appropriately noted, for the benefit of your child and the other children in family child care or in a center, your sick child will need to stay home until she is well and you will need to find an in-home substitute or stay home yourself.

Children need to be excluded from group child care settings when they have significant fever (>100.4 for infants 6 months and younger; >101.5 for older infants and toddlers), vomiting, diarrhea, pneumonia, significant asthma flares requiring frequent respiratory treatments, bacterial conjunctivitis or pharyngitis (drippy eyes or a sore throat), or a rash that is contagious, such as impetigo (bacterial skin infection).

Although juggling work responsibilities is challenging and many employers are not as understanding as we would like, an occasional day home caring for your sick child is an important part of parenting and offers a moment of quiet nurturing. Sometimes children, just as adults, are too ill to participate in their daily activities and need to stay home. Creative families have dealt with this in many ways: a family member may help out, or an at-

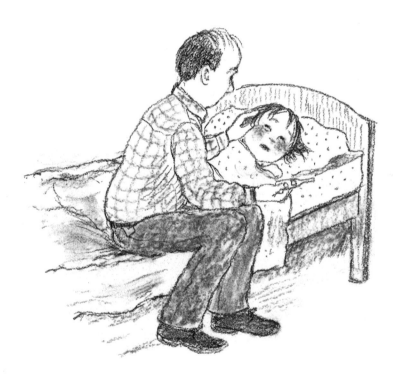

home neighbor might be willing to provide a day of care for a sick child in exchange for you providing evening child care so he or she can have a night out.

Some employers offer flexible benefits, where parents' sick days can be used for either their own illness or their child's. Whatever form of child care you ultimately choose, it is important to think through what will happen when your child gets sick so you have a plan you can put into place rather than scrambling for alternatives late at night with a sick child. For those of us who face snowy winters, think ahead about "snow days" when schools, preschools, and day care centers may be closed and back-up child care may again be needed. I know a few savvy working parents who have negotiated to have those days off ahead of time so they don't have the stress of the last-minute scramble.

Discuss ahead of time with your provider how to notify her and what to do when the child returns to the child care setting. In some cases, it may be appropriate for your provider to ask for a note of explanation from your pediatrician. In most cases with common viral illnesses that resolve with time, your child may be cared for at home and a visit to the doctor or nurse practitioner may not be necessary or appropriate. Fever is an important part of the body's defense system and actually helps kill the bacteria or virus that is causing the illness.

Because of the immaturity of their immune systems, minor fevers in young babies (less than two months) may indicate a serious infection, so a temperature of 100.4 or greater in this age requires medical evaluation. For older children, treat fever with acetaminophen or ibuprofen to lessen their discomfort with a higher temperature (>101.5) but don't worry too much about those smaller fevers. Avoid aspirin in children because of the risk of triggering Reye's syndrome, a rare but life-threatening condition involving the liver. Be sure always to check with your pediatrician about the correct dose of antipyretic medication (fever controllers) at each well-child visit, because the dosage will increase as your child grows older and bigger. After family, your caregiver is the most important caring adult in your child's life. Remember to be considerate of your caregiver and think about ways to show how much you value his or her efforts.

Open and honest communication with your caregiver is essential to maintain a healthy relationship with her, just as it is for all the other important relationships in your life.

A holiday bonus or birthday gift is lovely, and caregivers should always be compensated for extra hours outside of the regular schedule you have agreed on. The provider or child care center who takes care of logistics in a businesslike fashion and cares for your child in a loving fashion is a wonderful gift to a busy working family and should be treasured.

CHAPTER 4

Is There Something Different about My Baby?

When You're Worried There's a Problem

Today, many parents have busy schedules and live hectic lives juggling work and family. I may spend as much time with their children as they do. No wonder that on many occasions, I'll be the first to notice that something isn't quite right with a child.

Several years ago, I was shaking a rattle while playing with two seven-month-old infants, when I noticed something out of the ordinary. One baby was alert to my every movement, following the rattle with eye and head movements as I moved my hand. The other remained completely passive, seemingly unaware that I was shaking the rattle until I brought it close to her face. That evening I told her parents about the incident and suggested that they should have the baby's vision and hearing checked as soon as possible.

After an examination, their concerned pediatrician referred them to a pediatric neurologist, who found that the baby's head circumference was abnormal. After a number of tests and examinations, the baby was diagnosed with a rare congenital (inherited) syndrome that included vision and hearing loss, developmental delay, and other physical problems. She was fitted with tiny eyeglasses and a special hearing aid.

This girl stayed with me until she was four years old and then began attending a special school. While she was in my care, I had to be careful to make sure she didn't hurt herself. She liked to sit rocking back and forth, often near a wall, making "ah hah!" sounds. I was always afraid she might hit the back of her head. At first the other children in our group would laugh at her, but in a short time they came to accept and look after her in a loving way. Several years later when I saw her at a family occasion, she gave me a big hug and said school was "awesome!" The last I heard, she graduated from college, learned to drive, and was looking for a job.

I have cared for other children with diagnoses of a variety of congenital syndromes. Sometimes the parents were fully aware of the diagnosis when they first met me. Some of these children would stay with me for just a short time before starting school in an integrated special needs preschool. Others stayed with me longer, and I found the other children to be warm and accepting of any differences.

I have found that all children love books, even long before they learn to read. When I read a story, the children will sit in a circle, giving me their full attention. They also love to look at books, studying the pictures and making up their own stories. This is why I thought it was strange when one of the children showed no interest in looking at books or listening to stories. I told his parents that this seemed odd; later, when he went to school, the child was diagnosed with dyslexia. He had exceptional artistic skills, though, so dyslexia didn't stand in his way from attending an excellent college.

When our daughter was only two months old, her doctor told us that she had a "lazy" eye, for which she would be treated at the Massachusetts Eye and Ear Infirmary for several years. After attempting unsuccessfully to correct her vision by patching her normal eye, the problem was surgically corrected when she was three and a half years old. We still have a picture of her smiling broadly with a patch over her good eye, next to a snowman, which also had a patch over one eye!

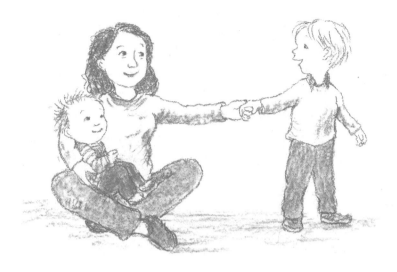

Because of our own experience, I am especially aware of the "lazy" eye condition and have alerted several parents to the possibility of a problem, advising them to have the child's vision checked. I tell all my parents that children should have their vision screened regularly by their pediatrician, with a referral to an ophthalmologist if there are any concerns. With early detection, most problems can be corrected easily.

Ear infections are a common complaint. I have mentioned to many parents that their child has been fussy and has pulled at an ear throughout the day. This may be a sign of an ear infection, so I will suggest that they take the child to their pediatrician for an examination. Nine times out of ten, the parents come back telling me that I was right, it *was* an ear infection.

Most of the problems I've seen were easily corrected. One girl cried whenever she had to put on her shoes. The solution seemed simple enough: swap her hard leather shoes for a softer pair. Her doctor did say, however, that the child had a minor orthopedic problem that could require surgical intervention if she didn't outgrow it. Fortunately, with time, the child seems to have outgrown the problem.

I like to report each child's progress on a continuing basis. When possible, I arrange for a longer than usual chat with parents at least once a week, scheduling time before or after their work. This is also an opportunity for parents to record the child's progress in their baby book. Beyond their sentimental value, such books can be a helpful record for future medical intervention. I tell parents when baby has discovered her hands, rolls over completely, sits up by herself, says "mama" or "dada," and, most exciting of all, takes those first steps. I've cared for several generations of children, and most of them were perfectly normal, arriving at each of these events according to Nature's perfect schedule.

I remember Peggy gently asking if anyone had ever noticed that my daughter's eyes looked a little crossed! Several appointments down the road, you can imagine that this pediatrician mother was horrified to discover that her four-year-old daughter had significant amblyopia (loss of vision in one eye) and mild strabismus ("lazy" eye). Thanks to support from Peggy, her preschool and kindergarten teachers, and her own wonderful determination, she now has near normal vision in *both eyes*, including remarkably good depth perception after a prolonged period of patching her normal eye. It was a good reminder to me as a pediatrician to continue to listen carefully when parents and caregivers express concern that something is not quite right with a child.

Peggy so beautifully describes the key elements to understanding and following a child's development: careful observation, comparison to the expected ages when certain milestones are reached, and seeking professional evaluation when a parent, grandparent, or observant caregiver has a concern. As parents we all want to believe our children are perfect and are often unaware of signs of a problem.

Routine well-child visits with a pediatrician, pediatric nurse practitioner, or family medicine physician includes careful review of a child's developmental progress, including sensory development, motor milestones achieved, and, of course, vaccinations essential to protect children from life-threatening infectious diseases. Bringing a list of questions to your child's checkup is a wonderful idea, because you will then remember what you really wanted to ask in the midst of a busy office. Reviewing the range of what is normal with your pediatrician is always helpful.

Developmental milestones occur normally across a range of several months, and each child progresses at his own rate.

Special circumstances such as prematurity or genetic syndromes such as Trisomy 21 (Down syndrome) will alter these milestones by several months. Children who fail to achieve a milestone within the expected range may be observed clinically for a period of time. If they do not show signs of progress, further evaluation—by Early Intervention (a state- and federally funded early childhood assessment and support program available throughout the United States), a developmental pediatrician, a neurologist, vision and hearing specialists, and other qualified professionals—will be warranted. If available in your area, choose pediatric specialists, especially in the evaluation of very young children. In areas of the country far from specialized services, try your best to find generalists who are experienced in evaluating children. We can all agree that children are not simply little adults!

If your child's medical caregiver or teacher is unresponsive to your concerns, don't give up. Feel free to call your child's doctor to discuss your concerns after your appointment. Your pediatrician may need time to reflect on what your true concerns are after your appointment and outside the hectic office atmosphere. Keep asking, look for a referral, or go for a second opinion until your question is answered and you have the information you need about and for your child.

Even with significant impairments or disheartening diagnoses, I always encourage parents to push for answers and information, which can empower them to act in their child's best interests. Negotiating the network of special education services in your community (available to all children at age three through federal Chapter 766 legislation) can be bewildering. In this arena, parent support groups and family advocates can be invaluable. The Internet has been a great resource to many families, helping them to locate parent support groups, more information, and specialized resources.

Parents are their children's best advocates.

And finally, each child is different, even when they carry the same diagnosis. I always tell parents to encourage their children, gently but enthusiastically, to do their best. Children derive great satisfaction from succeeding in whatever way they can. High expectations in a nurturing setting both at home, with your caregiver, and later in school will always serve your child best, no matter how their developmental progress unfolds!

CHAPTER 5

What Makes a Family?

Finding Your Own Way

What makes a family? In my experience with my own family, child care group, and extended circle of friends, I've encountered many varied family groupings. I have learned that one thing is certain about the makeup of a family: "one size *doesn't* fit all," in number, composition, or the values the members hold dear.

I grew up in a family of twelve children; my husband, Richard (Dick), was an only child of parents who had separated. After his mother died when he was a young boy, he was often cared for by his grandmother. Later he lived with his father and a stepmother. My mother also died when I was a young girl, and we younger children were brought up by our older sisters. It can't have been easy for them, as my eldest sister was only eighteen when Mama died.

I suppose you can say that certainly neither Richard nor I grew up in the kind of family we would see illustrated in the old "Dick and Jane" Elson-Gray Readers during our school days back in the 1930s. The brother and sisters shown in the books' pictures seemed to live an idyllic life in a tidy suburban neighborhood with a mother, father, and family dog, Spot. Some of the first words we learned to read were,

"See Dick. See Dick run!"

"See Jane. See Jane run!"

"See Spot. See Spot run!"

Of course, I have known some families who did fit the "Dick and Jane" model of American family life. I've also known and cared for children from many other types of families. I've cared for several babies adopted internationally by single mothers who wanted their children so intensely that they traveled to the four corners of the earth to bring them back to Cambridge. Adopting children from all over the world is becoming more common in our neighborhood as well as throughout the United States (see chapter 6). I've had several children who lived in two homes, as they were cared for jointly by their divorced parents. I've also cared for children with stepparents and who live with siblings from the parent's previous marriage. And, happily, I know many children who are well cared for in families with two daddies or two mommies.

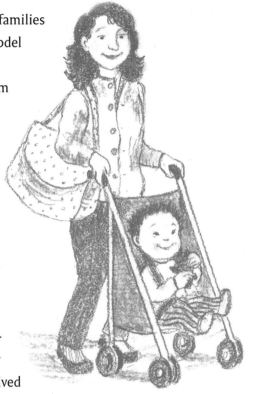

I like to tell people I've cared for children from every continent except Antarctica. The children come to me from a variety of cultures and religious faiths: Jewish, Muslim, Catholic, Buddhist, Protestant, and some families who don't follow any religious traditions. The children come from all different ethnic backgrounds, and for many families a language other than English is spoken in the home. Some families have been vegetarian; others have kept kosher households.

In every case the children in my care have always quickly accepted newcomers to the group—and people we meet on the street—as friends. Within my home we are all part of a "daytime" family. When you think of it, isn't *family* who you live with and love? If childhood is a happy time, family is always the place we later want to go home to, if only in our dreams. Sadly, for some children who never have a loving family they may wind up seeking companionship and unconditional acceptance from gang members and others in unsafe, unhealthy groupings.

When any of the children in my day care group talk about having celebrated a special holiday with their family, I always tell the rest of the children something about the holiday that is so important to their little friend. Children should learn about and respect each other's cultures. They learn by the example of their parents also respecting and celebrating the world's diversity of ethnic groups and cultures.

I suppose it was easy for us to teach our children to be tolerant growing up in as diverse a city as Cambridge. Here you often see people wearing ethnic or religious clothing such as an Indian sari or a Muslim hijab (head scarf). Having grown up in this community, my own children are comfortable traveling anywhere in the world. The United States is changing and becoming even more diverse with the arrival of immigrants from all over the world.

I believe that a child's first and most important lessons are learned from their families at home, where they learn both love and tolerance from the examples set by their parents and siblings. The second most important lessons are learned from their relationship with other children, in child care or preschool, and later at school. Unfortunately, some children, whose parents teach prejudice by their own examples, may try to influence your children later. As that wonderful song from *South Pacific* says of prejudice, "You've got to be taught . . . you've got to be carefully taught."

It is essential that, rather than prejudice, tolerance and compassion be carefully taught. If in your family life you show respect for everyone from all cultures, your children will learn that first and foremost. Other influences, including other children who may not have been as carefully taught, won't matter as much.

Parents are the first, best, and most important teachers of what matters most: tolerance, compassion, and respect for all.

Peggy has shared her wisdom on many issues that relate to creating the kind of family you want and how to emphasize some of the values that matter to you the most. Remember that you are not necessarily limited to following the path your own family followed. By choice or circumstances or a combination of both, many parents find themselves raising their children in a very different fashion than they themselves were raised. In every case, it is helpful to cherish the best of family traditions from the past and also to be inventive in creating new traditions that fit your family as it grows.

Today families often live far apart and can't always be together at holidays and milestone events such as christenings and graduations. Many parents deliberately create a family of choice to supplement their family of origin and invite friends to create holiday traditions together.

Many young parents need guidance in creating family structure, especially if they were raised in a fashion that no longer meets their needs or fits with their beliefs. For example, many parents who were disciplined with corporal punishment as they were growing up are strongly opposed to continuing this method with their own children. They need to be mindful in learning new ways of disciplining their children. Books, friends, and advice from your pediatrician can all be helpful if you are far away from your family or if you are choosing a different path from the one your family took.

If you are lucky enough to have grandparents nearby, cherish them. The relationship between grandchildren and grandparents is special indeed, as we discuss in chapter 20. Older aunts and uncles can fill a special niche as well if they are nearby, and family friends can be "chosen" as aunts and uncles. Children benefit enormously from having a number of loving, caring adults in their life.

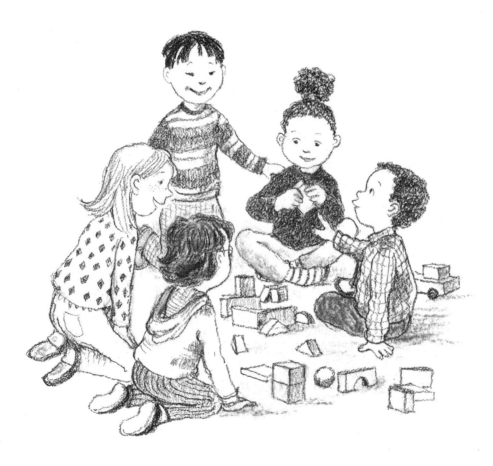

Children who live in two households do best when their parents set aside the conflict that led to the divorce and instead agree to work together for the children's best interests. Children should *never* be put in the middle or used to relay messages between parents who can't communicate with each other. It is imperative that divorced parents behave as grown-ups and set the right example for their children. The children will be most comfortable with a clear, easy to understand schedule and time with both parents if both parents are willing and able to care for them.

As with other challenges in life that young children face, reading stories on the topic of divorce can help them process their feelings. In *Dinosaurs Divorce*, Laurene Krasny Brown and Marc Brown use humor, clever illustrations, and a collection of endearing dinosaurs to help children make sense of the changes in their life when their family is in the middle of a divorce.

At a time when much in their world is changing, children will find routines comforting and reassuring, including knowing exactly when they spend time with each parent. Their schedule and pattern of going back and forth between homes will and should vary according to the developmental needs and ages of the children. As they get older, it is important that children have a say in a realistic fashion rather than being dictated to. Depending on the laws of the state where you live, they may even be able to choose which parent they want to live with at a certain age.

Children in single-parent households will also benefit from caring relationships with other adults, relatives, or friends. In fact, one of the key predictors of a child's success later in life is that they form at least one strong relationship with a caring adult: parent, teacher, coach, boss, or other role model.

Children in gay and lesbian households, raised by two fathers or two mothers, may face special challenges from the outside world, but their life at home is very much like the life of a child in a home with two parents of opposite sexes. Similarly, if their parents separate, the problems are much more the same than different from those of children of divorced parents of opposite sexes.

There is a growing body of scientific literature that confirms that children need the same from their families, no matter how family is defined. Love, limits, caring, unconditional acceptance, and the warm assurance that home is where you will always be loved are essential for children's health.

CHAPTER 6

If You've Chosen Your Child

Growing Your Family through Adoption

As a day care provider, I never experienced any difference between the needs of adopted children and those of the other children in my group. Each child has needed the same basics of love, limits, and nurturing, all of which I have delighted in providing. Still, because I enjoy keeping in touch with families long after their children outgrow my play group, I'm aware of a few challenges faced by adopted children after the preschool years.

One very big difference that I've noticed over the years is that adoption is now discussed openly, and this seems to be mostly a change for the better. Years ago, the fact that a child was adopted was kept a secret, sometimes even for life. Today, most parents are honest with their children, telling them at an appropriate age that they were specially chosen to be part of their family when they were adopted. For most children, it seems that parents start to tell them at age two or three, so they understand their family well by the time they go to kindergarten.

I've always been impressed with the extensive efforts the adoptive parents willingly put forth, with months of interviews, home visits, and even international travel to bring home a new baby. One mother carefully described the months of joyous anticipation and preparation as her *invisible* pregnancy.

She redecorated a room, picked out baby clothes, and sought out a highly recommended child care provider—me. As a single woman and busy working professional, she had to make many changes in her life to get ready to take on the exciting but daunting responsibility of becoming a new mother. Her child was a joyful addition to our play group for a number of years.

I've cared for many children who seemed to accept the story of their adoption happily. For some children, however, it seems to unmask deep fears. For example, one little girl developed a serious phobia about eating when told the elaborate details of her birth mother's history. Her parents sought help from a child psychologist, who helped her resolve this issue. Now a recent college graduate, she is pursuing a promising career.

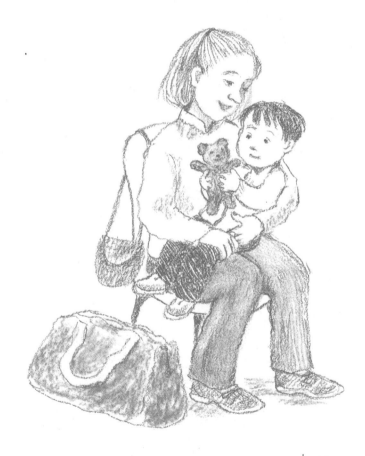

When to tell children they were adopted is a challenging decision that depends on timing. When a friend's daughter learned as a teenager that she had been adopted, she became upset and went so far as to take a name from her country of origin and even stop speaking to her parents. She remained angry for several months, until she came to appreciate how wonderful her parents were and how much they loved her.

Dick and I also knew a couple who adopted their niece and nephew from Europe, after the children's parents were killed in an accident. The children arrived at a young age and had to adapt to both a new family and a new country. We remember a story their father told us. One sunny fall day, about a year after arriving here, the father and daughter were walking back to Cambridge. They had just seen a Harvard soccer match, and were crossing the Charles River on a bridge close to Harvard Square. The little girl, now nine, reached up, squeezed her father's hand, and gave him a big grin. "I will always remember the day," our friend recalled. "I knew then we were truly father and daughter."

I'm happy to say that all the adopted children I have known over the years are living happy well-adjusted lives, even if there have been a few bumps in the road along the way. Children just need the basics and the knowledge that they are very much wanted and loved.

Adoption has become more common over the years, with 1.4 million adopted children, according to 2001 census data. Perhaps you are considering adoption for your own family. Or maybe a relative has just brought home a new baby from overseas or a neighbor is considering the adoption of an older child. Even if your children arrived via the more traditional biological route, he or she will certainly know adopted children as friends and playmates.

Over the years, I've cared for many adopted children from a variety of families. Some have been international adoptees, while others are local children placed for adoption by the Commonwealth of Massachusetts. Some have two parents, and some have one. Some have siblings who are also adopted, some have siblings who are the parents' biological children, and some have both. The one characteristic these families all have in common are that they have been created very mindfully. These parents truly wanted these children and for a host of different but equally valid reasons chose the route of adoption to grow their family.

Despite the differences in the families they have created, there are a few themes in common to all adoptive parents and their new children. Whereas biological parents have a well-defined term of pregnancy during which they can prepare for the arrival of their child, the experiences of adoptive parents vary widely. Some wait months to years, during which time the concept of that baby becomes very abstract. Others get a call shortly after completing their agency's requirements and leave the next day, with the nursery still unpainted and nothing ready for their return.

Every adoptive parent I know has said something similar to "the moment I held that baby in my arms, I knew she was my child." The combination of the trials and tribulations to get to that point, with the anticipation and excitement of finally meeting the child, help the parents bond with the baby immediately. For the children, the bonding is more gradual, depending on their own circumstances and ages.

The adoptive children who bond most easily with their new parents are those who have been in a single foster home until being adopted. They have had the experience of a consistent caretaker with whom to bond, and this helps them transfer that affection to their new family. Some do go through a period of mourning the loss of their foster mother, but this is a healthy demonstration of their capacity to emotionally connect with a caretaker.

Children who have been in an orphanage will need special understanding from their new parents. They are more likely to have had inconsistent caretaking and less emotional nurturing and, so, may be slower to form new attachments. Older children who have spent a long time in an orphanage, in particular, may be quite wary of new people, and siblings may be fiercely protective of each other.

Whether the adopted child is an infant or an older child, all children need enormous amounts of love, patience, and understanding from their new parents. Because they may be slower to reciprocate that affection, the emotional rewards may be slower in coming to the parents. Just take a deep breath and remind yourselves and the impatient relatives that "we all need time to adjust."

You and your child will have had many changes and transitions together, possibly even traveling across many time zones. Try to plan to take as long an adoption leave as possible to give yourself time to get to know each other before jumping into the busy complicated life of working parents juggling careers, small children, and child care. Three to six months is ideal. This might not be financially possible for some, but it gives you and your child the gift of time to adjust and bond before the child has to go through the next transition of adjusting to child care or a new caretaker.

The transitions will go more smoothly if you start to establish routines with your new child right away, even while traveling. Parents often pack a little stuffed toy or soft blanket to serve as the baby's transitional object while spending time traveling and in hotel rooms and airports. Thinking through and then implementing a bedtime routine is very helpful as well. For older children, pick a favorite bedtime story to read together every night, to start to establish your own routines.

Take lots of pictures during your travel and in the first few days with your new baby or child. Later, you can assemble them into a special scrapbook, journal, or video chronicle to document the beginning of your life together. Children love to pore over these special books that explain the beginning of their lives with you. There are also some wonderful children's picture books about adoption. *Tell Me Again About the Night I Was Born*, by Jamie Lee Curtis and Laura Cornell, is an imaginative, whimsical book about adoption which is very appealing to young children and their parents.

One of the things you will want to do during your first few weeks together is visit your pediatrician. Children who are international adoptees will need some special attention to their immunizations and screening for infectious diseases such as hepatitis B and tuberculosis, which are less prevalent in the United States. If your pediatrician has not had much experience with internationally adopted children, ask for a referral to an adoption clinic or travel medicine specialty clinic at a major medical center. Children born in the United States need a careful evaluation as well, because they may not have had consistent medical care during their early years.

Your pediatrician will also carefully assess your child's growth and development. The medical assessment of children from other countries varies widely. Some arrive with complete and accurate records, while others arrive with incomplete or even falsified information. Be sure to have all the information reviewed carefully and consult with a specialist if needed.

Children may arrive with undiagnosed heart murmurs, infectious diseases, or nutritional deficiencies that need attention.

Depending on the adequacy of the food available to your child before you met, her growth may not be optimal. Some children are overfed and arrive in an obese state. Others are underfed or have been fed a diet low in essential nutrients and arrive in an almost malnourished state. Most adoptive children grow remarkably well after they start to eat properly, so I like to watch them carefully and see how they develop once they are here.

There are some considerations in developmental milestones as well. Depending on the stimulation available to them before they arrived, babies may vary developmentally quite widely. A referral to Early Intervention for a careful assessment and provision of needed services such as speech and physical therapy can be very helpful. Some children may need a referral to a pediatric neurologist or a developmental pediatrician. If true delays or problems are detected, the appropriate supports from an early age can make all the difference.

In most cases, babies really begin to thrive after they arrive and feel settled.

Food, sleep, and toilet training can present challenges to adopted children and others. Particularly with older children who have had to scrounge for their own food you may see food hoarding behavior and overeating. With time and reassurance, they will start to realize life is now very different and that there is plenty of food in their new home.

Older babies, especially if they spent time in an orphanage, may never have had the opportunity to try solid foods or finger foods. Their skills in chewing and swallowing will be delayed compared to those of other children their age. Introduce new foods and textures gradually, just as you would with a younger baby who is trying solids for the first time at age four to six months. Soon your child will be eating everything.

Similarly, they may never have had the opportunity to learn to use a cup. They may be very tied to their bottle for comfort even at an age when most children are ready to give up their bottle. If that is the case with your child, begin to introduce a cup for drinking during the day, to gradually diminish his reliance on the bottle.

Because bottle use promotes dental caries, try to shift to a cup at an appropriate age. Avoid letting the baby drink milk periodically throughout the night, which also fosters tooth decay. Help your baby get used to drinking a bedtime bottle, having his teeth brushed, and then offer him water during the night if he needs to drink for comfort. Eventually you do want him to give up his bottle, but that will be something he truly clings to for comfort in the beginning of your life together. When he's more at ease and secure in his surroundings and with his new parents, you can work with him to get rid of the bottle.

Sleep is often a key issue for adopted children, particularly in the early days of their lives with their new families. Beyond infancy, children have to be secure and fully relaxed to fall asleep. Many children who have been in orphanages will have developed the skill of hypervigilence in self-defense and will lack an easy ability to nod off. Trying to fall asleep may stir up all their separation anxieties, and they may become even more awake as they are unhappily screaming in their bed.

You can take many steps and provide numerous cues to your baby or young child to help her become a good sleeper. A soft night light in the room will provide a visual cue at bedtime and is helpful to orient her when she wakes up. Pick the softest, fluffiest stuffed toy or blanket to use as a transitional object during travel and after returning home. This will serve as a tactile cue at bedtime.

Auditory cues work for some, but not all, children. Some children enjoy a music box or tape of soft music as they drift off to sleep. Others are hypersensitive to noise and will find it too stimulating or distracting at bedtime. Older children may even do well with headphones later as a way to calm down and relax at bedtime or when they are feeling anxious.

As your child learns to be a good sleeper think of this time as a short, self-limited means to an end. Try to stick to set bedtimes and bedtime routines as much as possible to help your child settle in. If after two weeks your child still hasn't started to improve their sleep pattern, talk to your pediatrician for some additional suggestions. It may feel stressful, but it is in everyone's best interest that your child become a good sleeper.

If your child arrives as a toddler in diapers, don't be in a rush to potty train him. He will be going through too many transitions at the moment to tackle this challenge too. Wait until he is settled, then start to gradually introduce the concept by reading stories, letting him sit on a little potty chair and pick out some big boy underwear.

As Peggy has noted, the needs of adopted children are much the same as other children, with a few variations. Have faith in yourself and the initial drive that led you to adopt. Watching a number of parents with their new children get to know each other has been gratifying and fascinating for me as a pediatrician. I've learned a lot from them, about how best to encourage and advise other parents as they bond with their new children. Trust your own instincts, and know that very soon you will start to feel very much like a family.

CHAPTER 7

What's to Eat?

Raising a Healthy Eater

My husband says that food fights were a daily occurrence in the cafeteria when he was teaching in a middle school. There are no food fights at my house, though, because I stress safety and manners. Just before noon, I tell the children to pick up the toys because "It's time for lunch!"

During lunch, everyone—including me— sits together in a circle. With safety in mind, I don't allow the children to walk about with food and drink. The children know they are expected to be polite, treat each other with kindness, and not make a mess with their food.

When I began providing lunch and snacks, I followed a menu plan suggested by a state-funded nutritional program. Once a month, the program would send a nutritionist from their office to check my lunch menus. This visit was fun for the kids, because the nutritionist staged puppet shows with fruit and vegetable characters to encourage healthy eating.

A typical lunchtime menu at our house might be pancakes, sliced apples, carrot sticks, milk, and a cookie. We use small plastic bowls and "no-drip" cups for the little ones. When several children are at my house for a meal, I ask the eldest to help me pass out lunch. The child feels very special and is thrilled to do it.

Until a child is one, parents supply baby food and, of course, breast milk or formula. When I first began as a child care provider I used to ask all parents to provide their children's lunches. It soon became clear that this

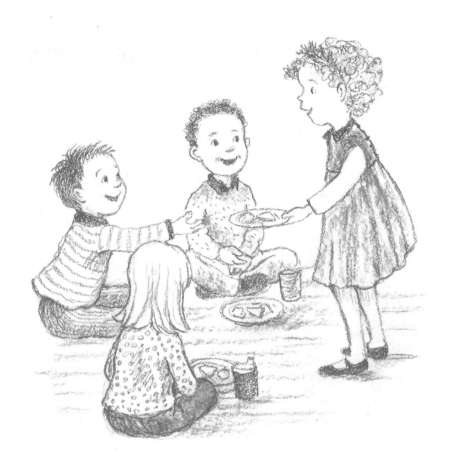

was a problem when the children invariably wanted each other's lunches. I decided it was best to provide lunch myself. It is easier when all the children (with the exception of those on special diets) eat the same thing. It is also an opportunity to introduce some children to healthy eating habits.

You would be surprised at what some parents allow their children to eat. This is usually because it is easier than saying no. I once cared for a child who often arrived with a lollipop in his mouth before having any breakfast. The parents had to rush off to work and couldn't spend any time fussing with Joey so he would eat something healthy. I didn't mind providing breakfast—usually toast, juice, and milk—but I wouldn't allow the lollipop in my house. More than one child has arrived at my house with candy before breakfast, but not recently. Today parents are more aware of the importance of good nutrition and establishing proper eating habits than in the past.

When possible, I like to allow the children to choose from my list of proven favorite lunches: grilled cheese, noodles topped with butter and grated cheese, or that old (and nutritious) favorite, a peanut butter and jelly sandwich. Each child gets a turn to choose the day's lunch menu, and, usually with some coaxing, the others agree. We also have tuna salad sandwiches, an occasional hot dog, "creamy" (cream cheese on toast or bread), pancakes with maple syrup, and applesauce or fruit slices and animal crackers for dessert. For mid-morning and afternoon snacks we have carrot sticks, apple juice, milk or water, and vanilla wafer cookies.

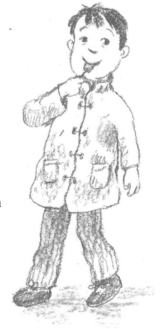

Parent-child control issues often emerge around eating. Years ago, I cared for a child who came to our group only twice a week. Her parents were surprised that she happily ate lunch at my house with the other children. The mother told me that the amount of food consumed during the child's time at home wouldn't add up to one bagel. Although the mother probably exaggerated, the child's eating habits were becoming a serious health problem and impairing her growth. The recommendations of the medical team evaluating this child included coaching the parents on how to avoid power struggles over food.

I think it is easier for me to avoid struggles over food with any child because I represent a different type of authority and may also present meals differently than some families. At my house, I make one meal for all the children, sit down with them to eat, and expect that we will have a pleasant meal time together. The children respond to these expectations and meal time usually goes smoothly. The peer pressure of the other children happily eating also has a positive influence on any reluctant eaters.

Some children require special diets. Parents who keep a kosher kitchen bring all of their children's food to my home. A few children have been vegetarians. If allergies are a concern, parents provide me with a list of the foods to avoid. Peanut butter and nuts are increasingly common and serious food allergies. If one child is allergic to peanuts, I do not serve peanuts or peanut butter to the group. I have cared for children who were lactose intolerant and for a child with an intolerance of wheat (gluten-sensitive enteropathy). Her mother baked bread and cakes using rice flour from Boston's Chinatown.

Speaking of special cakes, I can say with some pride that I make birthday cakes for children to take home on request. This practice started years ago when I made a theme birthday cake in the shape of a sailboat for one of the children. When the other children realized she was taking the cake home, they asked whether I could make them cakes to take home, too. It became a tradition beloved by me and the children.

In addition to sailboats, I've made cakes in the shapes of a train, cat, dog, clock, mermaid, and the ever-popular dinosaur. For one little girl I made a cake decorated to resemble a soccer field. The dinosaur is the only cake I make using a special pan; the others I construct by cutting and reassembling ordinary shapes into fanciful ones. Making the birthday cakes is both fun and my personal way to express love for each child. In my opinion, a day care provider should both care *about* children and care *for* children. Making cakes is one way I show I care about the children in my care.

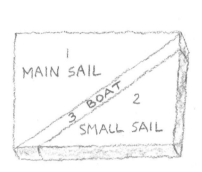 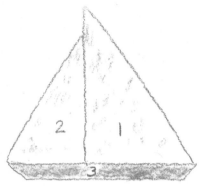

Cut cake diagonally in half, forming two triangles (labeled 1 and 2 in the diagram). From triangle number 2, cut a 2-inch strip (labeled number 3 in the diagram) parallel to the first cut. Arrange pieces to make a sailboat.

Peggy's Sailboat Cake

1 stick (1/2 cup) butter at room temperature

1 cup sugar

2 eggs

2 cups unbleached all-purpose flour

1 tablespoon baking powder

1 teaspoon salt

1 cup whole milk

1 teaspoon mace

Preheat oven to 350 degrees. Mix dry ingredients in mixing bowl. Add butter, milk, and mace directly to dry ingredients. Stir until smooth. Add eggs and beat by hand for two minutes. Pour into a lightly greased 11"x 14" rectangular pan and bake for 45 minutes. Assemble as directed and frost as you like to decorate your sailboat.

I remember a delicious and delightful sailboat cake that was a joy for my son on his third birthday. Peggy has described many of the tools required to raise healthy eaters: offer healthy choices, eat together as a family, model appropriate behavior at the table, and encourage the children to progress with their eating and serving skills in a developmentally appropriate way. We want to encourage our children to be confident, adventurous, and healthy eaters. Food plays an important role in all families and cultures. Under the best of circumstances, mealtime is a warm, nurturing time when families can connect at the end of a busy day. Under more challenging circumstances, it can become a frustrating battleground for children and parents alike.

Infants do best when fed breast milk for the first year of life. The many benefits of breast milk to the baby's health have been clearly established. Breastfed babies are healthier and smarter and are less likely to grow up to be overweight children. Families, caregivers, employers, and pediatricians should do everything possible to support breastfeeding mothers and their babies.

The beneficial effects of breastfeeding are indisputable for babies who are partially breastfed as well as for those who are exclusively breastfed. Babies are remarkably flexible and resilient, and they adapt well to a combination of bottles and nursing if that is what is required with the mother's return to work. Mothers who wish to continue breastfeeding should think through their return to work, their daily schedule at work, and their commuting time and then plan feeding along with their caretaker. Often a care giver can hold off on that late afternoon bottle, so that the mother can arrive and nurse the baby before heading home—a lovely way to reconnect after a day apart. There are many good resources to help nursing mothers. Above all, it is important not to become overly concerned about what and when the baby is eating. Pumped breast milk stored for the caregiver is wonderful, but supplemental formula is a nutritious alternative if the mother is not able to pump much when away from the baby. Nursing babies always love to nurse most of all. Babies should be fed breast milk or iron-fortified formula until one year of age.

Fortified infant cereal is another nutritious source of supplemental iron, which babies need by the time they are six months old. Introducing solid food is not only fun but also an important milestone for both parents and babies. Children who have a strong family history of food allergies and atopy (a tendency toward eczema and allergy) do better if they are not introduced to solid foods until they are six months old. Other children may be ready to start solids a little earlier. You will know that your baby is ready when you notice that she is very interested in what you are eating, when she isn't satisified with only nursing or a bottle, and when her tongue-thrusting reflex has disappeared and she can eat off a spoon. Because it introduces solids too early, takes away use of the tongue and lip muscles that is essential for speech development, and contributes to overfeeding and later obesity, adding solids to the baby bottle is not a good idea.

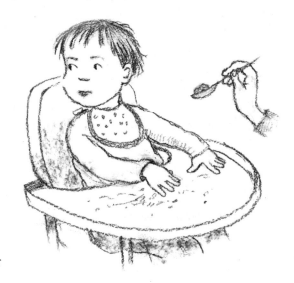

Always follow your baby's cues. When he is full, he will turn his head away. No need to "force" a child to eat at any age. There is new evidence to suggest that babies who are offered green vegetables on a spoon before the sweeter fruits and orange vegetables grow up to be better vegetable eaters later in life. And, remember, some babies take as many as twenty exposures to a new food before accepting it, so the first face at the first taste of green beans definitely does not mean he doesn't like them. He's just taking a little longer to get used to the new taste.

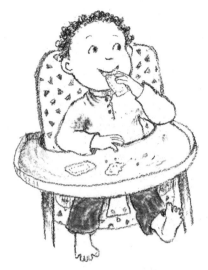

Offering a baby ages six months and older "finger foods" is another important milestone that parents and babies alike enjoy. Babies "practice" bringing their hands to their mouth first. When they have mastered that skill and can handle some textured food such as cereal, it is appropriate to start teething toasts and other foods they can hold and gnaw on. Miniature bagels are ideal. Starchy foods are best, because the baby's salivary enzymes will help to break down any pieces the baby breaks off. Later, soft pieces of cheese, tofu, bananas, avocado, and other foods can be cut into small pieces and the baby can help himself off the highchair tray.

As they try to make sense of their world, toddlers look for sameness and predictability. This preference for predictability applies to food as well as to other areas of life. Many toddlers go on eating "jags" when they eat a very limited diet. As long as they eat some fruit or vegetables, a source of protein such as an egg, fish, or chicken, and a source of calcium such as milk, cheese, or yogurt each day, they are probably doing fine.

Juice is a trap for babies, toddlers, and parents because children can fill up on the sweetened beverage and not eat other foods. Think of juice as a treat, not a nutritional essential. Children should get in the habit of drinking water from an early age and should have no more than four ounces of juice a day. If obesity is an issue, you will have to eliminate juice almost entirely from your child's diet. Children need the extra fat in whole milk until age two. After that, low-fat or skim milk is best.

Check with your pediatrician about the need for vitamin supplements; they are helpful "insurance" for the picky toddler who eats a limited diet. With encouragement, toddlers will outgrow the picky stage and expand their repertoire of food choices.

This is the age when power struggles over food can emerge. Your toddler's drive to be independent can assert itself at mealtimes. This drive can even supersede her sense of hunger. A fiercely independent toddler will refuse food even when hungry if pushed and cajoled too much. Parents can unknowingly exacerbate this situation by trying to feed the toddler just to make sure she "just eats something." It is easy to see how parents encouraging bites of this or that, and toddlers becoming increasingly obstinate and refusing to eat can turn dinnertime into a battleground.

If this sounds familiar, take a deep breath and rethink mealtimes. Your toddler has a short attention span and can only sit at the table for 10 to 15 minutes. Make sure everything is ready before your family sits down. Offer small amounts of a few foods on the toddler's plate and only one new food at a meal. Encourage your toddler to feed himself. After 10 to 15 minutes, let him get down even if he hasn't eaten much. He will be hungry later and eat more at the next meal. Try to avoid letting your child snack and graze continuously between meals. Three meals and two small snacks each day are plenty.

Preschoolers are just as curious about food as they are about the rest of the world. This is the age when children love to learn about food, help with cooking and shopping, and pick new foods to try. Consider fast food to be special treat, not a frequent staple in your child's diet. We all love it, but the additional salt, fat, and caloric content isn't healthy. On the other hand, an occasional meal at a favorite chain can be a fun break for everyone.

The most important elements of healthy, happy eating with children are

» Breastfeeding is best for babies up to one year of age.

» Advance your baby's diet as is developmentally appropriate.

» Never force feed a child of any age.

» Be patient, and keep trying new foods.

» Encourage water as the beverage of choice between meals in children older than one.

» Limit juice to two ounces each day for children ages one to three and to four ounces each day for children over three.

» Include five servings each day of fruit and vegetables.

» Offer whole grain products whenever possible.

» For the picky child who refuses the family meal, offer one acceptable alternative, such as yogurt, a bowl of whole grain cereal and milk, or a sandwich. The family cook should not have to whip up many different meals for different family members.

» Serve child-sized portions on the plate to help children avoid serving themselves too much and to prevent future problems with obesity.

» Enjoy food together as a family.

Helping your baby, toddler, or preschooler vary his diet as he grows and learn to love healthy choices in a relaxed, fun way is an essential part of parenting and will help ensure life-long healthy growth and development.

We now know that nurturing healthy eating habits in young children can lessen the risk of diabetes, heart disease, and cancer later in life. Helping your child learn to stop eating when full, avoid overeating, and eat lots of fruit, vegetables, and whole grains will give her a great life-long nutritional foundation.

CHAPTER 8

Don't Eat the Peanut Butter

Dealing with Children's Allergies

Not all good foods are good for everyone. Many children love a peanut butter and jelly sandwich cut into small squares. For many children, though, peanuts in any form must be avoided. When I interview new parents one of the first questions I ask is, "Does your child have any allergies?" Often allergies are related to food, and, because I provide lunch, I need to know what foods need to be avoided. Some times, of course, parents just don't know. I had such an experience myself years ago.

We were traveling on an ocean liner, when our four-year-old son had his first Coke. He didn't like the chalky-tasting milk served on the ship, so we thought a soda with his lunch would be fine. Soon after drinking about half a glass his lips became swollen and tender. We immediately sought medical attention at the ship's infirmary. The ship's doctor told us he probably had an allergic reaction to some ingredient in the soft drink. Treated with the appropriate medications, he was back to normal the next day, laughing and playing with his sister in the pool. I don't think he's had a Coke since.

When I know that allergies are a concern, I ask parents to provide a list of the foods to be avoided. Because my lunches are simple and don't contain likely offenders such as shellfish, it is easy for me to meet any child's special needs.

Today people are much more aware of healthy eating than was the case in the past. Most large supermarkets carry organic produce and prepared foods and a wide variety of foods formerly found only in specialty shops. It's hard to believe now, but when my husband and I were first married pesticides were considered quite beneficial to be used to promote crop growth. Then again, in those days cigarette ads featured doctors and athletes promoting the relaxing effects of smoking.

The adage "You are what you eat" holds true. It's essential to know that there are no harmful hidden ingredients in the food you give your child, especially when allergies are a concern. I've also noticed that product labels are becoming clearer all the time in carefully spelling out ingredients, but parents need to *read* the labels.

Surprisingly, I have never cared for children with hay fever (seasonal allergies) or asthma. These are potential problems a caregiver has to be prepared for in advance. I understand that a severe asthma attack can be life threatening. It is vital that your child care provider be given all emergency phone numbers, so parents and the child's pediatrician can be reached if necessary. With the widespread use of cell phones, most parents are easily reached throughout the workday.

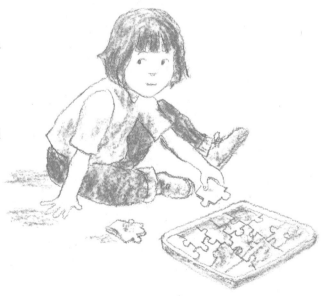

I have cared for a number of children with bad cases of eczema (atopic dermatitis). I have noticed that all the siblings in one family I've cared for have eczema. This is not surprising, because there is a genetic link. For the most part their mother applied the necessary topical treatments in the morning before dropping the children off, but occasionally I would apply the medications during the day. All four children outgrew the problem by the time they started kindergarten, but I've learned that not all children do.

Most children do very well despite significant allergies as long as they have the appropriate treatment. It is essential that everyone involved in the child's care—parents, child care provider, teachers, babysitters, and other family members—be well informed about the nature of the child's allergies and remain aware of the child's special requirements.

Allergies are a significant concern for many families. For reasons that are not entirely clear, the incidence of allergies, especially to food, in children is increasing. Allergies to peanuts are rapidly increasing, perhaps because there are traces of peanut in many prepared foods and children are exposed to peanuts incidentally as young babies. It is important for parents to be aware of what to do if their child is found to have a food allergy and for all parents to be aware of the signs of a first-time allergic reaction. These could be hives, swelling, difficulty breathing, vomiting, blood in the stool, or wheezing.

The timing of the introduction of solid foods is important to consider whenever allergies are suspected. For families with a history of food allergies, asthma, and eczema, delaying the introduction of all solid foods until the age of six months is beneficial and helps prevent the development of food allergies.

For all families, introducing new foods one food at a time allows parents to see whether their baby has a reaction to anything new.

There can be minor reactions to food that are not true allergies, but food sensitivities. Examples of these are rashes around the mouth after eating foods such as tomatoes or strawberries. If your child experiences a reaction like this, avoidance of that food until the age of two is a good idea; then carefully try it again after reviewing it with your pediatrician.

More severe reactions to foods are true allergies, triggered by specific antibody to a particular food or individual component. Examples would include hives (urticaria) after eating shrimp and facial swelling and difficulty breathing (anaphylaxis) to peanuts. Anaphylaxis can progress to a full respiratory arrest in which a child stops breathing. It can be very difficult to discern the difference between a food sensitivity and a true food allergy, so it is essential to review any food problems with your child's pediatrician. If there are any concerns, he or she may refer your child to an allergist to sort out the issues.

Once an allergy is identified, the role of the parents and other adults caring for the child is to make sure the child avoids this food. As Peggy mentioned, reading product labels is essential to make sure that products do not contain ingredients that need to be avoided. Meals at day care, restaurants, and at the homes of friends and family need to be carefully reviewed for your child.

Older children become quite adept at avoiding the foods they are allergic to, but younger ones will need your help. School-age children will find their school nurse a useful ally in helping to avoid foods in the classroom and the cafeteria. Children who are allergic to peanuts should sit with friends at a "peanut-free" table where all children do not bring peanut butter or any other peanut products in their lunches.

In cases of food allergy such as a reaction to peanuts, a preloaded syringe of epinephrine known as an EpiPen® is prescribed. This is something that must travel with the child at all times, to day care as well, in the event of a life-threatening allergic reaction. It is a safe, easy-to-use life-saving device.

You should be sure that you know exactly how to use it and that your child care provider knows as well. The pharmaceutical company supplies inactive models to use for training which are very useful. It is critical to remember when using an EpiPen® to call 911 and have your child seen in an emergency department within fifteen minutes of using it. In some cases there is a delayed second part of an allergic reaction even more severe than the first. Above all, stay calm if your child experiences an allergic reaction. Children fear shots and this is a very big one, so make sure you have other adults hold your child down firmly while administering the EpiPen®.

Antihistamines can be used to treat very mild, nonsystemic reactions. Be sure you have clarified with your child's doctor when and if you should give an antihistamine first or whether you should proceed directly to using the EpiPen®. Your caregiver will need clear instructions as well.

The diagnosis of an allergic reaction can be challenging for families of young children. With careful preparation and planning, you can be ready should a reaction occur and feel prepared to care for your child no matter what they eat.

CHAPTER 9

Time for Bed

Just a Sprinkling of Fairy Dust

After lunch is finished at 12:30 p.m. the children get their pads and blankets. I cover them up, sprinkle them with "fairy dust," and tell them to think happy thoughts. I begin by saying "ice cream." Each child calls out a thought or special idea: "teddy bear . . . birthdays . . . Mommy . . . goldfish!" It's just like a scene from the movie *Mary Poppins.* Children may toss and turn a bit, but soon become quiet, and within 15 minutes or so, at most half an hour, they are asleep. Many children happily follow the routine and nap here, even if they don't nap at home.

Parents ask about sleep, especially if their child rebels against bedtime or refuses to stay in bed, wanting instead to climb in with his parents. I can only advise them based on my experience with my own children when they were young and with the many children I've cared for over the years. Going to sleep readily is a learned behavior, and bedtime routines help children know what to expect as they get ready for sleep.

It is important to have a specific bedtime and a structure to the end of the day rather than just letting children fall asleep exhausted at any time. Children like routine. When my daughter was in the second grade, she wanted to know what was *her* bedtime? We didn't have a time set in stone, but we put her to bed after we finished supper and she played with her daddy. When she went to bed, either Dick or I read her a story before she went to sleep. Because her playmate had a precise bedtime, she wanted

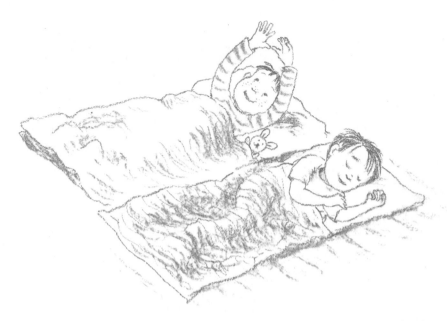

one, too. "Okay, then, you can go to bed at 7:30," we told her, and she did. That was about the time we put her to bed, anyway, and of course we still read a story first.

Going to bed should be a happy time. Every evening, as he sensed bedtime approaching, our son would ask how much time was left before he had to go to bed. When I told him "another two minutes," he would use up the time by continuing to ask me if his time was up. He is four years younger than our daughter, so during the preschool years he went to bed first. Our children were always happy to go to bed. They both looked forward to their stories and special time with us.

I advise parents to establish a bedtime they find appropriate and to remain consistent. It is best for the routine to be established at an early age. I realize this sounds like a simple solution to the bedtime problem. Frankly, it shouldn't be a problem. Just relax, stick to your routine, and enjoy putting your child to bed. Read to her or tell her a story, then say "Think happy thoughts" as you tuck her in, and, finally, kiss her "good night."

Peggy has noted the important factors in helping your child sleep well. Sleep is a family problem: when a child isn't sleeping well, often no one else in the family is sleeping well.

Tired parents are not at their best in the middle of the night trying to lull a baby back to sleep or lure a preschooler back into her own bed. No one can fault them for trying the easy way out and letting the child climb into bed with them. The best way to help a child learn to sleep well is to start at an early age, find routines that work for your family, and stick to them.

Doing the right thing to encourage good sleep habits is also the most difficult.

Children require different amounts of sleep at different ages. Infants sleep 12 to 14 hours each day, so the baby who takes several long naps of two to three hours during the day is not going to need to sleep more than eight to nine hours during the night. If the baby is sleeping during the daytime, and it has been more than two hours, wake him up. He is only going to sleep so much during a 24-hour period, and you want the majority of that to be during the night.

It is definitely acceptable to wake a baby up to shape his or her sleep; this will help the baby get on the right track to good sleep habits. Newborns sleep for short periods during the day and night initially and then gradually lengthen their nighttime sleep and condense their daytime sleep into several naps. Exposure to sunlight and fresh air, even in winter, is an effective way to encourage babies to sleep more at night.

Helping the baby learn to go to sleep on her own rather than being nursed or rocked to sleep is also helpful. Instead of waiting until she is completely adrift in a deep sleep, try putting the baby down gently when she is drowsy from nursing or drinking her bottle. Pat her gently if she rouses, and let her get used to the sensation of falling asleep on her own. Later, when she is able to sleep longer periods without eating, she will be able to go back to sleep on her own, rather than needing to be nursed or rocked back to sleep even when she isn't necessarily hungry.

Because breast milk is easily and quickly digested, breastfed babies will often need to nurse in the middle of the night long after bottle-fed babies are sleeping through the night. Helping an older baby learn the routine of waking up, nursing quietly with just a night light, and no stimulation or excitement and then going right back to bed helps everyone sleep longer.

Where should children sleep? In many countries and cultures the practice of cosleeping—that is, the baby sleeping with her parents—is common. Although this is certainly convenient for a nursing mother, co-sleeping is not recommended because it increases the risk of SIDS (Sudden Infant Death Syndrome) for a number of reasons.

Parents can unintentionally roll onto their babies. Babies can get stuck in tiny spaces between the wall and the bed. Also, adult bedding and bed surfaces are not designed for infants, who can't roll or barely lift their heads. The safest place for babies to sleep is on their backs, on a flat, firm surface such as a crib or bassinet. For parents who want the baby close to them, the bassinet can be placed adjacent to the bed. There are also cosleepers or sidecar baby beds available that attach to the side of the parents' bed, keeping the baby close by for nursing.

Toddlers sleep an average of 12 to 14 hours/day, usually with one to two naps and a lengthy nighttime stretch. Routines at nap time and bedtime help toddlers know what to expect and how to make sense of their world. Even very young babies can enjoy looking at a picture book of children's faces cuddled in their parents' lap before they are nursed and put to bed, and stories are an important clue for toddlers that bedtime is approaching and it is time to calm down.

Toddlers who still need to take a bottle or nurse before bedtime should also brush their teeth before falling asleep, because sleeping with a mouthful of formula or milk will lead to dental caries and the need for substantial dental work at an early age. Until children are coordinated and motivated enough to spit out the toothpaste, just moisten the toothbrush with warm water but no toothpaste and use the brush to mechanically clean the surface of the teeth. Most children enjoy brushing their teeth, but a few determined toddlers need limits set about the importance of teeth brushing twice a day as well. Toothbrushes with bells or music are a big help, and going right to a fun activity such as a story immediately after brushing is a good distraction.

Toddlers who have temper tantrums at bedtime are often overtired or don't have enough of a routine to help them predict what is happening next. Slowing down the pace of bedtime or starting a half hour earlier may be helpful. Moving bath time to evening and using it as part of the calming down routine can also help.

Toddlers are not at the most flexible stage, so this is a time when parents can't be as mobile as they might like. Especially with traveling, hosting visitors, welcoming a new baby, or other big changes in routine, sticking with

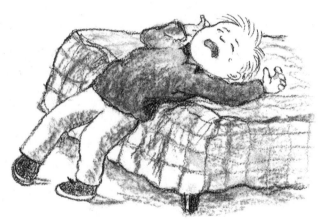

a toddler's regular bedtime routine and schedule is vital to helping a little one cope with changes and face his world well rested.

When do children outgrow their naps? Every child is different. Some are done with naps at two to three years old, and others still need them when they get to kindergarten. Some may give up naps temporarily and then need them again during a significant developmental milestone such as toilet training or starting preschool or kindergarten. Even when they no longer need to nap, a quiet interlude when the child is calmly on her bed with favorite animals and books for 20 to 30 minutes is a nice way to slow down in the middle of the day.

Preschoolers need to sleep 11 to 13 hours every day. The child who has outgrown his nap is often ready for an early bedtime. This is the age when magical thinking and fantasy begin to play a large role, so children might be preoccupied with monsters in the closet and sounds in the night. As with many issues, children can often work out their fears through stories. *Bedtime for Frances* by Russell Hoban and *Max's Bedtime* by Rosemary Wells are tested favorites, along with the Margaret Wise Brown classics *Goodnight Moon* and *The Runaway Bunny*. Preschoolers can often concoct elaborate ruses and distractions at bedtime such as "just one more drink" that require parents to be firm and reinforce the usual limits and routines.

It is in everyone's best interests that children sleep well. We know children are happier, better adjusted, and even grow better when they are well rested. Certainly their parents are better rested when the children are sleeping well. Think carefully how to help your baby, toddler, or preschooler "learn" at each stage how to sleep well. In the end, you will help everyone in the household get a good night's sleep.

CHAPTER 10

The Crying Baby

What Does She Need, and When to Worry?

"It has been a nightmare!" our friends said when we went to their house for dinner years ago. The new mother was holding their howling, red-faced infant.

"Believe me, we have tried everything. Our pediatrician says that Sally has colic. We take turns walking her during the night—sometimes all night. The only thing that seems to help a little is the hot water bottle we wrap in a receiving blanket and place against her tummy. The warmth seems to comfort her for awhile."

We felt so sorry for our friends. This was before we had children, and we wondered whether, when the time came, our own baby would also cry night and day. Later, when she was a few months old, Sally's painful colic simply went away, and our friends began to enjoy a happy family life.

Parents in my day care group have told me other stories, but I have no direct experience in caring for infants with colic. Most of the children I care for come to me when they are at least three months old, which I understand is usually beyond the colic stage.

Fortunately, none of the small number of younger infants I have cared for, as well as my own children and grandchildren, have had colic. The families whose babies were colicky said that nothing seemed to help and that they just had to make the best of those stressful months.

I've also heard stories of parents getting up several times during the night in response to a baby, who seems to cry only for attention. I recently took care of a fifteen-month-old boy who throughout the day played happily in our group and took peaceful midday naps with the other children. He cried only when I changed his diaper. Many babies fuss when being changed.

I was surprised to hear his mother would get up three or four times each night to comfort him when he cried. She said there was never anything wrong with him; he just wanted to be held. This is a common problem. As I often say, babies are smart. It doesn't take long for a baby to figure out that he can cry and then be picked up and held in a parent's warm and cozy embrace.

Often a baby does cry for a good reason, such as being hungry or thirsty or needing a diaper change. Sometimes a baby may be overstimulated by active play before bedtime or simply be overtired. In the case of the mother getting up several times a night to comfort her fifteen month old, his daddy and older sister loved to "roughhouse" with the little fellow before he was put to bed.

From my experience I would suggest that, if a baby continues to cry after having been fed, changed, and burped, it's okay to let him fuss a bit. After all, going to sleep is a learned behavior, and babies have to learn to fall asleep on their own.

I strongly believe it is important for babies and toddlers to have a regular schedule for feeding and sleeping. It doesn't have to be a rigid schedule, but generally sticking to the same times for feeding and naps is helpful. Similarly, during growth spurts babies will get hungry more often and need to be fed sooner. In general, babies and toddlers do seem more content when their lives follow a regular pattern.

It also seems that the temperament and emotional state of the parents will strongly influence a baby. An atmosphere at home that is anxious and agitated affects the baby. Tense, fussy parents may have a fussy baby, while in most instances calm, happy parents usually have contented infants. Colic is a major exception to this rule.

Sometimes a baby may cry because she is bored. I've observed that babies both enjoy and need visual images. Colorful picture books with different textures on the pages to touch are fun for babies and help them improve their motor skills. Some parents bring their baby's own activity or play gym to my house. These are useful items for keeping a baby engaged. He can watch a mobile or pull on objects such as stuffed animals and even listen to music.

Of course, you can provide the best entertainment of all by singing to your baby. Even if you're an off-key Judy Garland, be assured you can count

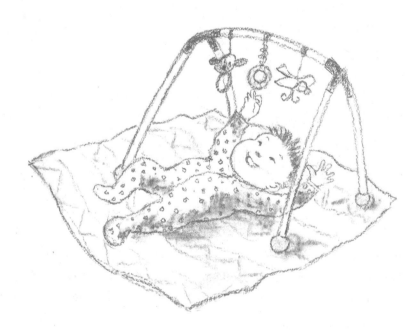

on receiving rave reviews. Your baby will think you're wonderful. Babies, toddlers, and young children all enjoy music, whether singing in the shower, whistling, or listening to recorded music.

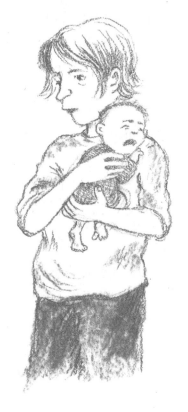

Every parent wants to know how long to let a baby cry under normal circumstances. With a newborn, you have to be the most attentive. You should respond immediately and make sure everything is all right. Most often the baby will need to be burped, changed, or fed. If everything is fine and you've tried to meet her needs in all of these ways, you can let her cry for a reasonable time, say 15 to 20 minutes, until she falls asleep. You may want to check on her from time to time and pat her gently. It's important to leave the baby in the crib, so you don't teach her that crying results in her being picked up.

When all is said and done, we can agree that under normal circumstances and at the appropriate time parents should welcome a baby's cry. After all, it's the only way a baby can tell us what he needs. A baby who doesn't cry can sometimes be a greater concern. We expect a normal healthy baby to cry from time to time.

I often hear of parents who are so accustomed to waking when their baby cries that they continue to wake even when their baby is silent. They slip out of bed to check on their baby and find her sleeping contentedly. Usually within a few days to weeks everyone adjusts to the new routine and is happily sleeping through the night.

Babies are uncomplicated beings. They usually cry for very understandable reasons: hunger, a wet or dirty diaper, a burp that needs to come up, or the need for comfort and closeness. Our job as parents with very young infants is to anticipate and understand these needs and meet them, to build trust and a secure sense of self in the infant. Erik Erikson articulates this so beautifully in *Childhood and Society,* where infancy is described as the stage where "trust versus mistrust" is fostered.

Consistently meeting a baby's needs helps him to grow in a secure fashion. Babies learn to trust, and trusting infants progress developmentally to be older babies who are able to tolerate a bit of frustration and who can be put down and amuse themselves for a few moments. Meeting a baby's needs does not mean that he or she has to be held constantly. There will always be times when the baby needs to be put down. A busy parent needs to take a shower, answer the door, make a phone call, or cook a meal. Gently placing the baby in his crib or playpen is the safest practice and helps him learn that it is just fine to be on his own for a bit and that you will be back.

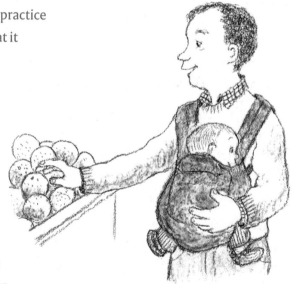

Babies enjoy the close comfort of being carried in a sling pack or front pack. They are snuggled in nicely and will often sleep in the pack, while you have your hands free to take care of things. On a cold day you can bundle the baby in the pack inside your coat to really keep her warm. Fresh air, even in the winter, helps regulate sleep cycles and calm the crying baby.

Helping babies stay amused and content also prevents or shortens crying spells. As Peggy noted, babies enjoy things to look at. Your baby will often sit contentedly in her seat watching you while you work in the kitchen or at a desk. Particularly if you talk to her from time to time and give her a rattle or other interesting toy to shake, she will do fine and enjoy being near you. Babies love watching faces, so placing a mirror nearby is a helpful technique. Babies with older siblings are fascinated by their older brothers and sisters and adore watching them do anything.

It is important not to be afraid of a baby's crying. As parents get to know their baby, one of the things they learn quickly is what different cries mean. A tired cry is different from a cry about a wet diaper, and both are different from the roar of a hungry baby. Pay attention to the different qualities of your baby's cries and you will find it easier to understand how to soothe him.

There is a normal progression in how much babies cry as they grow. The amount of time a baby cries gradually increases over the first month to its peak, about two hours total in a day, at the age of two months. From then on, it gradually decreases and becomes much more specific in response to actual events or needs. This also coincides with the time that the baby starts to spend more time awake and begins to show early signs of communication, such as smiling in response to a familiar voice or face.

As Peggy noted, there will be times when you've tried everything and the baby won't calm down. It is very reasonable to gently lay the baby down in a safe place such as her crib or playpen and step away for a moment to calm yourself down. Leaving the baby in a darkened room often helps to calm her as well. Pay attention to any feelings of frustration or anger you may be experiencing, because this can lead to the tragedy of shaken baby syndrome. This is when the force of shaking a baby can cause serious brain damage or even death. Never shake a baby for any reason.

After you set the baby down and step away for a moment to calm yourself down, you may return to find the baby asleep. If not, try unwrapping the baby and look him over head to toe. Look carefully for any signs of redness or swelling. It is easy for a hair to wrap around a tiny toe or finger, causing pain. Babies can also scratch their eyes and cause corneal abrasions. This is also a good time to check the baby's temperature, because sick babies are often very fussy.

If you've done everything, and the baby is still crying, try swaddling him tightly and carrying him in a pack or bundled up in your arms. If inconsolable crying continues for an entire morning or afternoon, it is definitely time to call your pediatrician, who may very well want to see the baby that day. Remember that babies who are overtired and haven't slept at night will often have trouble sleeping the next day. It's as though they are too tired to pull themselves together and calm down enough to sleep.

Another possibility is colic, a poorly understood condition of young babies. It is defined as periods of inconsolable crying in an otherwise well baby for more than three hours total per day, more than three days per week, and lasts for more than three to four weeks until the baby is about three to four months old. If your baby has long stretches of inconsolable crying, you will definitely want to visit your pediatrician because colic is a diagnosis made only after a number of serious conditions have been excluded.

Pediatricians and other researchers are still trying to understand exactly what colic is and what causes it. Most are in agreement that it probably is due to immaturity of the baby's nervous system, and also perhaps their gastrointestinal system, that leaves certain babies difficult to soothe and calm. It can be very stressful to new parents because colicky babies are demanding and certainly not much fun. These babies are notable in that their development and growth are perfect despite their periods of colic.

If your baby is diagnosed as having colic, know that it is a time-limited period of difficulty and that he will grow up to be a healthy happy baby after all.

Because so many factors can make a baby cry, the science of studying colic is complicated. There are a few interventions that have been shown to help some babies calm down, at least a little. They are the following:

» Being carried in a front pack or sling.

» Being exposed to white noise, such as the washer, dryer, or car noise, and vibrations.

» In some cases of formula-fed infants, a formula change to a formula containing hydrolyzed proteins after consultation with your pediatrician.

» In select cases of breastfed babies, eliminating certain foods from the mother's diet after consultation with your pediatrician.

If your baby has colic, this is a good time to take up your friends and family member's offers of help. Someone else can come over and watch the baby, even walk her or take her for a ride in the car, while you take a bath and relax or take a nap. Remember how helpful earplugs can be in these circumstances. Parents will have to work together as a team, working in shifts to get through the night with the baby and taking turns sleeping.

For single parents, colic can be especially trying and overwhelming, so don't hesitate to ask for help. The best thing about colic, experienced parents will tell you, is that it finally ends. The joy and relief at finally having a typically responsive baby is remarkable.

Whether a colicky baby who seems to cry endlessly, or a typical baby with normal amounts of crying, all parents are faced with the puzzle of a crying baby from time to time. If you stay calm, think through all the likely reasons for crying, attend to them all, and look at the baby carefully, you will undoubtedly find the answer to your child's cries. It is a very satisfying moment in parenting when your screaming little red-faced baby relaxes into a peaceful, calm, sleeping baby.

CHAPTER 11

I Have to Use the Potty

The Ins and Outs of Toilet Training

Toilet training is a frequently discussed subject among new parents. I've heard that some people have lifelong "hang-ups" concerning their own toilet training. That's unfortunate; happily, with the children I've cared for over the years I've never found it much of a problem.

I usually begin when the children are about two and a half years old, although some children are ready at an earlier age. I start by just talking with them for the first week about what to expect in the bathroom. I explain that they are growing up and are ready to use the toilet just like the big girls and boys.

I show them how the toilet works and describe what to expect when they sit on the seat. Some parents will bring a "potty chair" from home when I mention that I am going to start training, but I have never used one because I don't find it necessary. After a week of only talking about going to the toilet like big boys and girls, I begin by taking the children to the bathroom at 10:30 a.m. I show them how to sit and hold onto the toilet seat. At first, I only leave them for a minute, and chances are nothing happens. Before nap time, at 12:30 p.m., we repeat the process and try again after nap as well.

As with everything for children, keeping to a routine is very important. The training usually takes about a week before they get the idea and are able to use the toilet on their own. Good hygiene is emphasized at all times, with the children learning to flush the toilet and wash their hands when they are finished.

Praise and rewards encourage children. In every case I use abundant praise throughout the process. For some children, I keep a chart giving a gold star, along with lots of praise, each time they "perform." When more than one child is involved, the praise of their peers is often enough of a reward. When a child was first successful, we would all clap and cheer, calling out, "Hooray for Tommy! Good job!" Actually, it seemed somewhat easier training several children at a time because they encouraged one another. I once trained five children all at the same time. By the end of a week, after busily working together, most of the children were doing quite well.

Making a game out of learning to use the toilet kept it from seeming like a pressured situation for the children. It is a big thrill for all to see the "graduation prize," when the successful child gets to wear big boy or girl underwear. When they see this, the others are envious and eager to finish training so they can wear big kid underwear, too.

Going to the toilet is an act some children will use as a situation to control at home. They will cheerfully "perform" at my house and then regress to using a diaper at home. Why is this? My guess is that some children are like Peter Pan and don't really want to grow up, at least not too soon. After all, by then their long-time favorite, the bottle, is gone, and diapers represent the last trace of being a baby.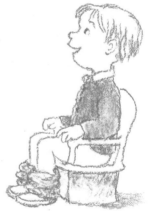

Success with bowel movements for some children comes earlier, but for some children they will literally "hold on" and refuse to have a bowel movement in the toilet for a long time.

I remember a perplexed mother who asked her son, "Why do you do 'brown potty' in the toilet at Peggy's, but not for me at home?" Again, I think it may be part of subconsciously not wanting to grow up and wanting to remain a baby for a little longer. It's understandable. All too soon it's time for preschool, and before long the children will be coming by to give me a hug before going off to college.

I imagine we would all have loved to see the commotion of five little ones busily being toilet-trained all at once. Children can be the best cheerleaders for each other, as they encourage each other to do more, better, faster.

Peggy's stories illustrate what is the most important principle of toilet training your child: motivation, and by that we mean the child's, not yours.

Children need to have achieved several milestones in different domains of development, in order to progress happily through toilet training. They need to be sturdy walkers and runners to get to the bathroom, and children with impaired or delayed mobility will need a sensitive caregiver who helps them get to the bathroom on time. They need the fine motor dexterity to get their pants down, so this is a good time to dress your little ones in sweat pants that are easy to get up and down. They need to have the verbal capacity to say, "I have to go, now," and neurologically they have to have achieved continence of bladder and bowel.

Continence, or the ability to hold urine or stool until is time to urinate or defecate, is achieved gradually, usually first with bowel and then with bladder. A young infant urinates very frequently, and, as she grows older, gradually has longer and longer periods of staying dry. Toddlers in the pre–toileting stage will often announce, "I'm pee-ing!" while wearing their diapers, and that shows they have achieved the understanding of what it means to have a full bladder and what happens next.

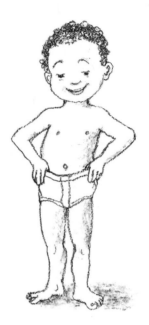

This is the time that children start to hide be-hind curtains or go off into corners for "privacy" when they are having a bowel movement. This also is a good sign because it shows that the tod-dler has an understanding of what needs to hap-pen, when they have that sensation of fullness.

The key to successful toilet training is to build on both your child's success in achieving these milestones and her desire to succeed and please you. "Pooping in the potty" for the first time can be quite an event, as Peggy has described. Make a big deal over all potty training successes and pay as little attention as possible to the failures. Try saying, "Oh well, I hope you'll use the potty next time."

You can enhance your child's potential for success by encouraging her to sit on the toilet after eating. There is a lot of normal intestinal move-ment, the gastrocolic reflex, which is stimulated by the process of eating, and it moves everything along in the digestive tract at that time. Many parents are very good at reading facial cues that might indicate "it's time" and gently encouraging the child to "try" the potty. Children also need to feel safe sitting either on the regular toilet with support and a stool for their feet or on a small potty chair where their feet can touch the ground, so they have full use of all muscle groups to void and defecate.

Achieving full bladder control, especially at night, may take longer. For newly trained preschoolers, an occasional daytime accident, when they forget to go to the bathroom because they are too busy and absorbed in play, is not unusual and certainly not a setback. Many three- or four-year-old children are dry during the day, wearing underwear and using the toilet for urination and bowel movements, but still need a nighttime diaper or pull-up to avoid nighttime bedwetting.

There is a strong familial component to bedwetting, or enuresis. It is more common in boys than girls by a ratio of three to one, so if your child has many uncles in the family who wet the bed, brace yourself. Most will outgrow it by the age of six, but at that age there are still approximately ten percent of children who have not achieved nighttime continence.

If your child is older than six and still wetting the bed, speak with your child's pediatrician about using special alarms or medications to help a child stay dry. Being a habitual bedwetter at older ages can take a toll on a child's self-esteem and impede his ability to participate in wonderful social opportunities like sleepovers and overnight camp. Most children who continue to wet the bed are not lazy or unmotivated but are very deep sleepers who simply do not register signals from their full bladder to their brain.

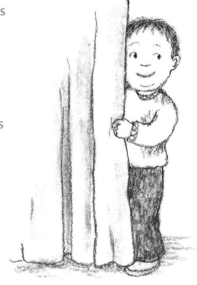

Toilet training can raise other issues for children and parents that you might need some help from your pediatrician as well. Picky eaters can often become constipated from a diet with few fruits and vegetables, and this can become a real issue around the time of toilet training. If your child is constipated and painfully passes a big hard stool, it is very likely that the next time he needs to go he will hold on to his stool to avoid the same thing happening again. This starts a vicious cycle of infrequent, large, painful bowel movements. The best way to avoid this is to make sure your child eats lots of fiber-rich foods like whole grains, fruits, and vegetables and drinks lots of water.

If you notice blood in your child's stool or large and painful but infrequent bowel movements, speak to your child's pediatric provider about this. He may need some help with a fiber supplement or short use of a prescription medication. Other issues to bring to your health care provider's attention include

» The child who was fully trained and then regresses.
» The child who seems to have no concept of his need to urinate or have a bowel movement by age three.
» The child whose urine begins to sting and burn.
» The older child who has been dry at night for years and starts to wet the bed again consistently.

These symptoms can all indicate a medical or emotional problem, and it is best to seek help early.

Aside from constipation, we do sometimes see a child who is simply not motivated to use the toilet. As Peggy noted, this may be a control issue. Remember that children at this age are striving to assert themselves and feel competent. It is essential that they are given a few choices in areas in which it is appropriate for them to make their own decisions: what to wear, what to eat (within reason), what toys to play with, and what piece of playground equipment to try first. With a reasonable amount of freedom to choose, children are less likely to stake out their control in areas such as eating and using the toilet.

Special events, such as an opportunity to swim in a pool or start preschool, can also be used as helpful motivators to encourage children to use the toilet and give up those diapers. Star or sticker charts can be helpful ways to provide positive reinforcement and chart a child's progress.

A reward can be special time alone with a parent at the end of a few good days. Fancy underwear the child has picked out is often a great motivation, too. Toilet training is a big event in your child's life. By understanding all the developmental and emotional issues involved, you can structure the beginning in a purposeful way and help your child enjoy success.

CHAPTER 12

He's Just Shy
Your Child's Temperament

I remember being shy as a little girl. I grew up in a time when children were expected to be "seen and not heard," and to be somewhat timid when introduced to strangers was considered normal behavior. We were expected to "speak only when spoken to" when we were among adults.

Aren't we all, children and adults alike, somewhat uncomfortable at first in new social situations? It's understandable that when children first join our play group they may cling to their parents and have a hard time separating from them. That's why I warn parents ahead of time that it's best to just give a hug and leave quickly than prolong the leave-taking.

The child may cry briefly, and this is as difficult for the parents as it is for the child. After we wave goodbye at the window, the child may want to be held for comfort. I tell concerned parents that they are welcome to listen at the door after they leave.

Usually they will hear that in less than a minute their child has stopped crying and is happily playing with the other children. The children are often remarkably sympathetic, offering hugs and pats on the back to the crying child.

A word about the physical surroundings in which children spend their day at my house may be in order here. I think of our place as a home in the truest sense. It is casual and comfortable and filled with photographs of children and the many places we have traveled, especially Italy and England, where we have family.

Most of the day's activities take place in my living room, where plastic boxes of toys are stacked next to a bookcase. I always sit in an old Boston rocker, which the children call "Peggy's chair." From here I watch and supervise the children's play. Parents have told me they feel it is a warm and child-friendly atmosphere.

I always ask a new parent to call back in about an hour after leaving my house, just to check in case the child does have difficulty adjusting to a new environment. If the child is crying inconsolably, I suggest the parent return and we try again another day. Sometimes the newness of the surroundings is simply overwhelming and the child may need to regroup before coming back the next day. Fortunately, this rarely happens.

Most children adapt quite quickly to a new setting such as child care, especially when given lots of preparation to get ready for the change. Within

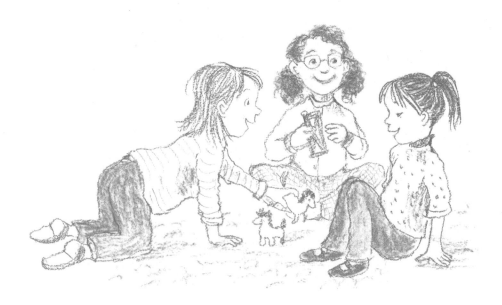

a day or two after starting with my group, new children are greeting their friends eagerly in the morning, waving goodbye to their parents, and settling right down to play.

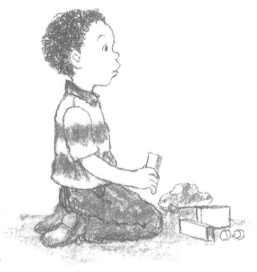

There usually isn't any separation problem with children who start with me as infants. We soon bond and I am accepted as an important part of the child's life. I have on occasion cared for an insecure baby who cries if I leave the room even for a moment to warm up a bottle.

Often when older, a shy child will be perfectly happy playing until other children's parents start to arrive at pick-up time. The insecure child may then move away into a corner, and seem timid and afraid, until his own parents arrive. Shy children will often be quite timid when they meet up face to face with Dick and me outside but holler from a distance, waving wildly from across the street.

I've also cared for more outgoing children. These are the children likely to greet everyone's parents with big hellos when they arrive. I like to encourage all the children and parents to greet each other and socialize a bit at the end of the day.

One mother told me she had to caution her child not to go with strangers because she was afraid her daughter would go off with someone. Her concern was understandable. Fiona was a delightful child with a sparkling, outgoing personality and a wonderful sense of humor. It is an unfortunate but realistic fact of life that happy, innocent children have to be taught that not everyone they meet is nice.

Some children find it difficult to adjust to a group. They may just be shy by nature. Most children happily play, side by side, until they are about two and a half and then start to actually play with others. Shy children may prefer to continue to play in a solitary fashion until they are older and ready to reach out to other children.

I once cared for a boy who asked to go off and play alone in my dining room because he wanted to be away from the other children. I encouraged him to stay with the rest of the children and reminded him he was a valued member of our daytime family and that we all enjoyed one another's company. That shy little boy is a young lawyer now, so he certainly grew up to become more comfortable dealing with others.

Although I like to encourage every child to participate in our play group, I also try to recognize and respect each child's individual temperament. Some children prefer certain toys every day, while others are eager to try everything in my toy boxes. Most get quite territorial and choose the same spot for lunch and naps daily. They like to use the same color plastic bowl and cup at lunch every day and always choose the same pad for their nap. Over the years, it has been quite a delight to see the variation in temperament among all my children. Every child wants to be respected, and certainly deserves to be, as the wonderful individuals they are.

Understanding your child's temperament can help you do a better job of supporting him. Most mothers will report they had a very clear sense of their baby's temperament from their activity level in utero even before they were born. Parents who adopt infants report that their new baby begins to declare her own personality as soon as she starts to feel at ease in her new surroundings.

Think about how your baby or young child handles a new situation.

Some babies are alert and interested in everything around them, from a very early age. Others are quiet and more content to watch from a corner or tucked in a front pack carried by a parent.

How does your toddler handle new situations? Does she rush right in and start exploring, or does she hold back and carefully survey the scene before making a move? Is he happiest in a crowd of children, such as a playgroup or classroom, or off by himself, playing in parallel with one or two other children nearby?

Outgoing and gregarious children may be eager to have new experiences but need more help from parents in pacing themselves in order to not become overstimulated and overtired. These are the babies that go until they drop exhaustedly for their nap and later as toddlers may resist taking a nap even when they still really need it. You can help by structuring your day to make sure there is sufficient quiet time to settle down before a nap or bedtime. These active children need more time for transitions at the end of activities because they are so intensely involved with what they are doing at the moment that it is difficult to pull away.

More inwardly centered or shy children will need time at the beginning of activities to observe, adjust, and get comfortable before

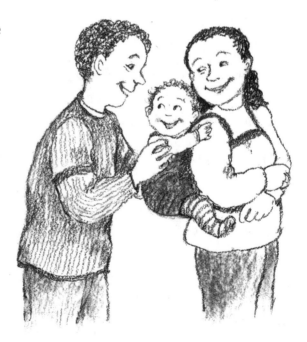

they join in or settle into a new play setting. Shy children may be quite friendly and interactive once they feel secure with their new surrounding and new playmates. All children like to know what to expect in new situations, and this is especially true for shy children. Reminders of the day's activities or what will happen next are also helpful for all children and help them adjust. Driving to or riding the bus to child care or another activity gives you a moment to review what happens each day with your children.

Your child's temperament can also help you to choose an appropriate child care setting. There are many factors that will have to be evaluated, such as suitability of the child care providers, hours of operation, and convenience but keeping your child's temperament in mind will be useful, too. All other parameters being equal, a shy child might do better in a small group setting instead of potentially feeling overwhelmed in a larger class in a child care center. A lively active child might thrive in the bustle of a larger facility.

Is the activity you have in mind suitable for your child's temperament? A lively, active child will enjoy a tumbling class, but a shy child might prefer a self-paced discovery activity at a local nature center. Parent-child activities or classes are good ways to encourage your child to try something she might not take to right away. As parents we want to help our children have a broad range of experiences.

How can you best help your child when he is in a challenging situation due to a mismatch between his temperament and the setting? First of all, make a decision about the flexibility of the situation. An enrichment class or fun activity should be just that, not a chore to be withstood. If the activity turns out to not suit your child, see about changing to something else or getting a credit to try a different class at another time. Most people dealing with young children will understand.

Sometimes there may not be much flexibility involved. For example, if you need a certain placement because of its hours and availability, you may not have other child care options.

Never offer a choice to your child if you are not in a position to make a change.

After reviewing the child's placement to be sure that there are no red flags about unsuitable or unsafe situations, try to help your child know that you see he is struggling and that you will do everything you can to support him. It is not a bad thing for children to learn that sometimes in life we have to make the best of a less-than-perfect situation. Speaking to the child care provider or center staff about ways to adapt the program for your child, within reasonable limits, can be helpful.

For example, a shy child may adjust more easily if paired with a "buddy" in her class or child care group. A very active child who is restless in a small family day care might be given special "jobs" that involve lots of running up and down the stairs, or extra play time outside if that can be accommodated with supervision. Children are remarkably resilient, and with some support from you and minor adjustments by the child care provider most children can adapt to situations that might at first seem daunting.

As adults we often find ourselves in situations that might not be in perfect harmony with our own temperaments, but we strive to adjust. Helping our children learn to be flexible and develop good coping skills will help them to succeed in a variety of settings regardless of their underlying temperament.

CHAPTER 13

No Hitting!

The Aggressive Child

At one time or another every child will do something naughty, such as hitting a playmate or grabbing a toy. I immediately correct the child, calling him over and making eye contact, as I ask him what happened. After he tells me, I want him to explain such actions, telling him, "It isn't good manners to behave like that. Now tell Lucy that you're sorry." At this point, the child usually begins to cry. Kids have a hard time saying "Sorry," so that is a punishment in itself. If he refuses to apologize, I send him to the corner for a "time out," telling him he has to stay there, until he says he's sorry.

Eventually all children do apologize. They are only in the corner for a minute or so. Some just take longer than others. After the child comes out of the corner, I ask the two children to hug, tell them "it's over," and they quickly resume playing.

I remember a child who would cut the process short by putting herself in the corner as soon as she grabbed a toy or pushed someone. She would then turn around and say that she was sorry.

I've had children who are happy all day but become aggressive at the end of the day when their parents arrive to pick them up. This can happen for any number of reasons. Sometimes children try so hard to behave well during the course of the day and as a result have pent-up energy to get rid of at the end of the day. Sometimes they are expecting one parent and the other arrives. This can be tricky because most children go through a phase of preferring one parent to the other.

When a child does ask me who will be coming to pick him up in the evening, I reassure them that it will be one or the other of his parents. Often with single-parent families a friend or relative may pick them up instead of the parent. In either case, I'm careful not to commit. Parents' plans can change throughout the day, and children have a hard enough time leaving. A tired, cranky child can easily fall apart at the end of the day and act out with a temper tantrum or aggressive behavior if surprised or dismayed by who is picking them up.

When I'm alone with the children tantrums are extremely rare. If it does happen, I find it best just to ignore the child, who, of course, is seeking attention by acting out. The tantrum will soon run its course, and the child will resume playing with the other children.

Kids don't like to be told what to do but instead enjoy structures that help them to know what to do. Often they fuss about putting on their coat, when parents arrive, even to the point of throwing a tantrum. For this reason, I like to have them get ready early, before the parents arrive, so they can leave on a happy note.

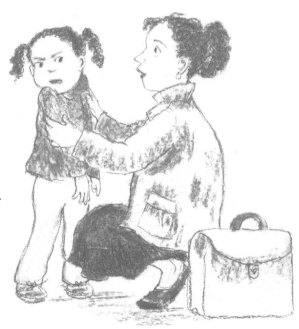

Are some children mean? I have seen mean or sneaky traits, which no doubt result from others having treated them in a mean way, and I suppose children learn dishonesty from adults who are not honest with them, but I'm reluctant to say that children can be mean.

Biting can be considered mean behavior, yet only once has a child in my care bitten another. This was a two year old whose mother said he had a bad weekend at home with his four-year-old brother. The mother warned me that the two year old was arriving that Monday morning with a lot of pent-up frustration.

Needless to say, I was very upset when he bit the one year old on his cheek. The children were playing together without any suggestion of a problem when the older child bit. Of course, I immediately called the child's mother to tell her that her child had been bitten. She was also very upset.

I also talked to two local pediatricians about the incident, and they told me it wasn't that unusual for children this age to bite. Sometimes children are testing limits, and sometimes younger children are just curious.

We once experienced the situation as parents, when friends were visiting us for a day during our Cape Ann vacation. For no apparent reason the visiting older boy bit our son. Maybe he was jealous and upset because he wasn't staying longer with us at the beach.

I once had a child whose aggressive behavior was encouraged by his father. As soon as he came in the door he would want to hit or kick the other children in my group. His mother told me that his father encouraged this behavior by rough play with him in the evenings. A small man himself, he wanted to ensure that his son, even at the age of eighteen months, would be a tough kid who no one could push around.

After his mother would leave, the child usually settled down nicely, but he always required close supervision. He could be very sweet and displayed a great sense of humor, but it took time for him to be fully accepted by the other children.

Over all these years, there has only been one child I've asked to leave my house. The little boy, a two year old, had been in multiple child care situations already and had many obvious anger issues. Although the mother warned me, I agreed to take him on a trial basis for three days. It was a mistake.

During the three days, he continually tried to hit and kick the other children. I had to watch him constantly. The poor child was obviously very unhappy, but, in fairness to the other children, I felt I had to tell his mother he just wasn't suited to our setting. I also encouraged her to seek some professional help to work on these problems, which would only get worse as he grew older.

Several parents over the years have told me it would be all right to spank their children if I thought it necessary. I would *never* hit a child because that isn't the way I care for children. Spanking isn't necessary; children respond nicely to love and limits. These little bursts of aggression, when handled promptly from the start, fade quickly and don't become big issues. The children in my care learn to behave with kindness and gentleness toward one another because that is what I expect.

Aggression in children is difficult for the adults around them to handle. It comes in two varieties. One is the type of acting out in an aggressive fashion that toddlers do. They may hit their parents or another child or even bite to see what happens. It's not an indication of deep-seated problems, just a stage that most little children pass through.

When this happens I encourage parents to speak firmly and loudly, in their sternest voice. "No biting in this house!" or a similar warning usually is enough to convey your disapproval and sometimes even bring on tears. While you certainly don't want to make your child cry, in this case you will know your message of disapproval has been received.

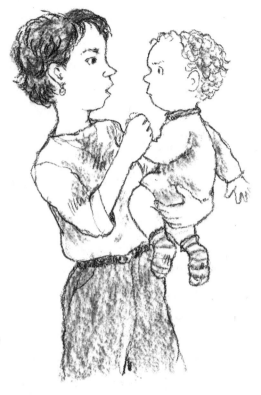

In many cases, when toddlers hit, kick, or bite, it can be kind of funny, almost comical. Try your best not to laugh, as that will certainly encourage this very undesired behavior. If young toddlers hit or bite again, after your stern warning, remove them from the situation, place them in their crib or playpen for safety, and say again, sternly, "No biting in this house!" Then walk away. Usually the combination of your stern warning, being removed from the situation, and the lack of your attention is enough to squelch this sort of behavior.

There is also a normal physicality of play that should not be confused with aggression. Starting with toddlers, most little boys tend to play with each other in a more physical fashion than little girls do. As they get older, wrestling and friendly punches are part of their play. These are neither aggressive nor intended to hurt or harm the others. Little girls' play patterns tend to be more communicative and collaborative, with more verbal sharing and passing back and forth of toys.

The second type of aggressive behavior that is seen with young children is when they develop a pattern of consistently acting out or responding to frustration by hitting, biting, or kicking others. This is upsetting to other children and adults. If this is a consistent response on the part of your child, it is a sign there is a problem. Perhaps another child is hitting yours and she is modeling that behavior. A caregiver may be disciplining in a way that is not consistent with your wishes. A child with significant speech delay may strike out when he can't make his wishes known. A child with an undiagnosed hearing loss may act out similarly.

Peggy and I share a similar belief in the absolute unacceptability of spanking as a way to modify the behavior of young children. The science of studying spanking is complex because there are many factors involved in parents' choice of discipline. The data on the use of spanking are used by both proponents and opponents of spanking to support their views, much to my dismay and those who also oppose spanking. However, one point is unequivocal. Spanking teaches young children that grownups around them can hit them, and that is not a desired thing to foster trust, love, and good behavior.

Whatever the cause of your child's aggression, you need to deal with it promptly. If responding to a few incidents of biting or hitting in the manner described doesn't stop the problem but instead you see an escalating pattern of behavior, it is time to get some help. Take a careful look at the surroundings in which your child spends his day and make sure that he is not modeling undesired behavior or that an adult caregiver is not punishing him by hitting.

Unsupervised television viewing can sometimes be the culprit. There are many things on television that are full of violent images, and young children have no sense of how to interpret them. They may be acting out something they've seen on television or the wrong kind of video and put-ting a stop to watching the wrong things can help improve their behavior.

Look carefully at the relationships among the older children and adults in your family. Children of all ages are very perceptive of violent behavior among the adults around them. If you are involved in a domestic violence situation, get help, for yourself and for your children. While these are very complex situations, we do know clearly they do not go away—they just escalate. The National Domestic Violence Hotline—1-800-799-SAFE (7233)—can connect to you to help and resources in all fifty states, twenty-four hours a day, year round.

If your older children punch each other and try to hurt each other, get help for them. A family counselor or therapist can be very helpful in look-ing at patterns involving the whole family. He or she can work with you together, help you understand the unhealthy patterns that trigger these responses on the part of various family members, and help you find new ways to interact with each other.

If, after carefully assessing your child's environment, you find nothing that is problematic, talk to your pediatrician or nurse practitioner about how best to help your child. They can help you with a more specific plan tailored to your child or refer you to a specialist if necessary. Sometimes a few sessions with a child psychologist or child psychiatrist can make an enormous difference. Identifying the problem is the beginning of solving the problem. It is a useful model that will serve you well no matter how young or old your child is. You will both feel much better knowing what the problem is, and how to solve it.

Getting help for your child when something clearly is not right is an essential task of parenting.

CHAPTER 14

Quit Picking on Your Sister!
Raising Siblings in Imperfect Harmony

My sisters and brothers always played an important role in my life. Coming from a large, close-knit family, I loved them all. While growing up I was closest to those nearer my age, especially my sister Rose.

She was only a year younger, and for a time we went to boarding school together. Naturally, we share many memories of childhood secrets and adventures. I still remember the day we skipped school to see a wonderful concert sung by a young Frank Sinatra. To this day, he is still my favorite.

I suppose it is true for many people: a sibling can be your best friend and someone you feel you can always count on when needed. In the case of my family, it was our two older sisters, Ellie and Irene, who took the place of our mother after she died. They did a remarkable job, caring for the nine younger children, for which we will always be truly grateful.

Children can learn many things from their siblings. My older brothers are responsible for my love of baseball. During summer Saturday afternoons, they would let me join them and their gang to share bowls of freshly made popcorn, while listening to a Red Sox game on the radio. Despite the absence of a Red Sox World Series championship until 2004, it was generous of them to encourage my love of baseball and share time with their kid sister.

Many years ago, I cared for a couple of free-spirited siblings, a five-year-old girl and her three-year-old brother. They were both mischievous and fun, and Dick thought they behaved like the impish characters "Thing One" and "Thing Two" in the Dr. Seuss's *The Cat in the Hat*.

To this day, the brother still holds the record for the most time-outs in the corner. When she was punished the brother became very upset, but when he got into trouble she couldn't have cared less and, in fact, found it to be very funny. In this case it was the younger child being more protective of the older one, although most often I observe it is the reverse. They both grew up to be delightful, accomplished young adults and good friends.

More recently I've cared for a brother and sister pair. Although they were two years apart in age—they were two and four at the time—they played together nicely. When the younger sibling needed help I would often hear the older say gently, "I can help you with that."

With the children in my care, I can say that the older children have always been kind and helpful to the little ones. Seeing each other every day and having to share toys with each other makes our day care group a little

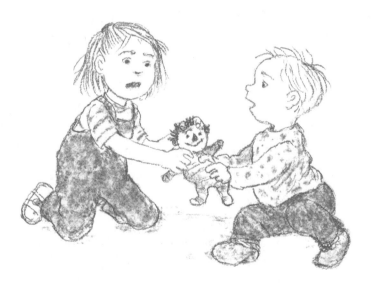

like an extended family of brothers and sisters. The children even compete for my attention, just as siblings do with their parents.

Years ago when our son was an infant and had a fever, I was holding him and applying a cool wet compress to his forehead for comfort. Our daughter, who was five years old at the time, asked, "Did you do that for me when I was a baby?" I told her that I did, and gave her a big hug. It's natural for a child to crave a parent's love and attention and even feel a pang of jealousy when the parent attends to a sibling. In our house there was little competition over clothes or toys because we had a child of each sex. Sometimes when we gave a special gift we knew both children would enjoy, such as a stuffed toy collie dog Lassie from the popular television show, we would put "To Share" on the gift tag.

My son can remember happy days alone with his mother when our daughter was in school. Of course, she also recalls the fun we had together before her brother was born. Although we continued to give her the same loving attention as we did when she had been an only child, the birth of her brother certainly was a big change in her life.

No matter how large your family becomes, it is important to try to give each child equal attention. It's not possible to give children of different ages exactly the same kind of attention, but the time given to each is important. Caring for a newborn is very different from playing with or reading to an older child, but both will thrive with your attention.

My husband was an only child, but he doesn't recall being lonely. Rather than playing with brothers or sisters, he had neighborhood kids and school chums to play with. His neighborhood pals were all about the same age and all boys. He admits, though, that he missed having an older brother to emulate or confide in or a younger sister to protect.

Sharing among the children in my family was never a problem. None of us had much more than the basic necessities. I can remember being delighted when I was given twenty-five pennies in a recycled candy tin for a Christmas gift. Those pennies seemed like a fortune at our local candy store. The younger girls in the family were always delighted to receive our older sisters' outgrown clothes and felt quite stylish and grown-up to be wearing them.

Although I have heard many stories of sibling rivalry, I've been fortunate with my own children and the children I've cared for over the years. Most of the siblings I've known in my child care have enjoyed happy, loving relationships that continued on into their adulthood. I credit the parents for having been sensitive to each child's unique needs and for nurturing these healthy sibling relationships.

The question of siblings is something about which all parents think carefully. Our families of origin have shaped our own childhood markedly, whether we had siblings or were an only child. Birth order also influences our childhoods. Parents may try to recreate their own family in terms of numbers of children, or may try a very different direction depending on the quality of their experience as a young child.

Unless your first pregnancy resulted in the arrival of twins or other multiples, the first decision you will face related to siblings is whether to have a second child. If your family began by the adoption of your first, you will be faced with the decision of whether to adopt a second child.

This is a very important and personal decision. Families in the United States have become smaller over the years for many reasons, including the shift to an urban society, economics, and two-working-parent families. While your friends and family will undoubtedly share their opinions, it is really only up to you and your mate.

According to the U.S. Census Bureau and its report *Living Arrangements of Children: 2001*, 21 percent of children live in households with no other siblings present. For many people, the decision to limit their family to one child makes sense. Family size and structure have been well studied and only children do just fine. The key to helping only children succeed is to include the child's friends at home often, in your daily activities as well as special outings so that your only child does learn how to take turns, share, and think of others as well as herself.

If you do decide to have a second child, or adopt a second child, you will want to consider the timing of that second child. Biologically speaking, it is optimal for the mother to wait about two years between pregnancies to let her body recover. Developmentally, some children have a difficult time negotiating the stormy waters of the second and third year, and the addition of a new baby at that time to cope with is taxing. Others sail right through. Older children, four and up, may be more secure in their own developmental progress and so are more eager to welcome a new baby.

Realistically speaking, the timing of that second baby may be subject to many factors: parents' own health, new jobs or educational programs, even natural or man-made disasters. For example, obstetrical departments nationwide experienced a baby boom nine months after the events of September 11, 2001, and again after Hurricane Katrina on August 26, 2005. If you are struggling with infertility issues, the timing of your second baby will be subject to the requirements of any reproductive technology you require. Adoptive parents have little or no control over the timing of the arrival of their children. If you are hoping for a second baby, the timing is what it is. You will do your best to prepare yourselves to parent more than one child and get your first child ready for the biggest change in his or her entire life.

The key is to prepare your child for the arrival of a sibling in a way that is developmentally appropriate to his age. Very young toddlers under the age of two have little concept of time but will be aware of your growing tummy. Children's ability to comprehend varies tremendously at this age, so you never know what they understand. It is appropriate to say something like, "There is a baby growing in Mommy's tummy, and the baby will be here in a long time."

For these younger children, the arrival of the new baby really is a shock. It is as if the infant dropped from the sky. Children of this age will need lots of attention from their parents and from their mother, especially when she is not nursing the new infant. This is an ideal time to take up the offers of help from friends and family. They can take the baby in between feedings, and you can be free for some special time with your first child. Your child will need lots of reassurance and lots of hugs and physical affection.

With children this age you want to work toward changes well in advance of the arrival of the new baby. For example, children who are rushed out of their crib or who have their bottles taken away a few weeks before the baby arrives are not very happy and tend to show a lot of regressive behavior. A child who has settled happily into her big girl bed a few months ahead of time will not feel like the baby has taken her place.

If your child is not ready to move into a bed, don't rush her. It will be much easier for you to have your older child stay in her crib and sleep well after the baby arrives than to be restless and pop up out of her new bed all through the night. The new baby will be perfectly happy sleeping in a bassinet, cosleeper, or portable crib for a few months until the older child is ready to ease into a big bed after the initial adjustment phase.

Similarly, right before your new baby arrives is not a good time to focus on toilet training for the older child. If he is not ready two to three months before the baby's due date, just keep two sizes of diapers on hand and wait until after the baby's birth and his adjustment to make a major push. Diapers are a big expense, but family members can help out by bringing you sizes for both children as gifts or doing a load or two if you wash your own. If he is just barely out of diapers when the baby arrives, all his testing and acting out may take the form of lots of accidents and needing to be back in diapers. This is an unhappy parent-child interaction and does not help him to feel competent and grown up at a time you really want to be able to praise him for his big boy actions.

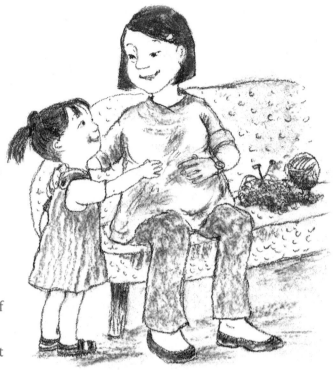

Older children of three and four can really appreciate and understand more of what is happening as they see their mother's tummy grow. They will be able to transfer their understanding of their friend's baby sisters and brothers to their own family situation. They are at a good age to help by bringing diapers, carrying a blanket, or choosing a stuffed toy for the baby.

Toddlers and young children should never be left alone with the baby. A frustrated toddler will sometimes poke at the baby, and children will often innocently give babies small toys or food like raisins or nuts that can choke them, so a grownup's supervision is essential. The baby can go in his crib for safety, and his older sister can come into the bathroom with you for company while you shower. It will save you time and worry in the long run.

Some children gain siblings through remarriage and the creation of a blended family after a divorce or the death of a parent. According to the U.S. Census data, 15 percent of children in the United States live in blended families, most often with one biological parent and a stepparent, along with children from both adults' previous marriages. Blended families provide instant siblings but a host of other challenges as well.

There are a few things that can help a newly blended family surmount those challenges. The parents need to be explicitly clear with each other about their expectations in terms of parenting each other's children. Some families will choose to have both parent and stepparent equally involved in parenting and discipline, while others will agree that each parent disciplines only his or her biological children. All models can work, but each requires patience and explicit communication.

Children in a blended family each need their own space and things. Ideally, moving to a new house or apartment as a new family helps everyone start out with a fair chance and equal familiarity with the new living situation. Each child needs his or her own room. If that is not possible and children share rooms, make sure that each child has designated space within the room for their own things.

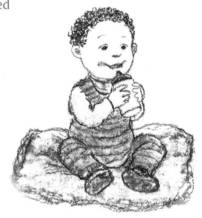

Children in a blended family also need some time alone with their biological parent on a consistent basis. They need and should receive lots of reassurance that even though things feel quite different, their parent's feelings for them have not changed and that they are still loved. A blended family can be the beginning for a wonderful new life together and can work well if everyone communicates clearly, tries their best, and keeps a sense of humor and perspective about the inevitable ups and downs.

Regardless of how the siblings come to live together, whether by birth, adoption, or blended families, many of the issues are the same.

Children need reassurance that they are loved, and they need that reassurance often. They are quick to sense inequity and injustice. Even very young children can sense when adults choose favorites, and they don't like it one bit. The most important thing that you can do as a parent to help your children live harmoniously together is to treat them fairly.

If we are fortunate enough to have siblings, we have a built-in peer group right at home, someone who shares our upbringing and childhood, and someone later in life with whom to share the care of our aging parents. Children can use their siblings to practice all sorts of things and better learn how to get along in the world. The arrival of your child's new sibling will be a big change in their little life, but you can be certain he or she will be a wonderful gift.

CHAPTER 15

Say "Please"

Good Manners in Young Children

Nothing will influence your child more than your personal behavior. I once knew a perfectly loving family whose members always seemed to shout at one another, even during general conversation. It's not that they intended to be rude; it was just their normal state of affairs. As a consequence, their children were always shouting.

If children hear their parents speaking in a polite, moderate tone, they will follow their example. When they grow up, good manners will be a natural part of their demeanor and will help them to be comfortable in every social situation.

Good manners *are* important. Sometimes it seems as though they have been forgotten. Courtesy simply makes everyone more comfortable in any social exchange. I'm a senior citizen and have trouble standing for prolonged periods of time. All too often, I have to ask someone to give me his or her seat on a bus or subway train. Some young people are thoughtful and will rise to offer me a seat as soon as I board the bus, but far too many of all ages choose to ignore passengers in need of a seat.

I wonder whether some teenagers are embarrassed to show good manners. Maybe they are afraid their peers will laugh at them, but both boys and girls seem reluctant to use good manners. In many television shows popular with teens and young adults today, many of the characters seem rude. They are constantly shouting and insulting each other against a backdrop of canned laughter.

No doubt the media, movies, and certainly school friends do influence a child's manners and behavior, but if manners have been carefully attended to nothing should negate the positive influence of a good home environment. As new parents, you are probably just beginning to realize how powerful an influence you have on your child. Your good example will serve your child well for a lifetime. I once met a woman who told me the greatest gifts her parents gave her were the ability to love well and be polite.

In my day care group, I constantly emphasize the basics of courtesy and respect to the children. I encourage them to respect each other and the parents who come and go daily. When children and parents arrive in the morning, I remind each child to say "good morning." It's one of my first lessons in good manners.

As new parents, don't be surprised when, even in a group, your young child will be content to play alone. Parallel play is the norm among children under two years of age. Don't worry that your child is antisocial. It is just normal behavior for this age.

Of course, most little children will grab toys from each other. After many gentle "no-no's" and being shown that grabbing isn't kind, most children learn how to behave. When they grow older and start to play together and exchange toys, I insist that they say "please" and "thank you" to each other. Of course, this isn't automatic, but with gentle repetition and encouragement, this small courtesy will begin to come naturally.

You don't need to, and really shouldn't, reward good behavior with a gift, but you should always praise a child when appropriate. Children often come to my house with a new toy that has been given for good behavior. This can be done for extraordinary circumstances but certainly should be the exception and not the rule. Gifts in exchange for good behavior begin to serve as bribes.

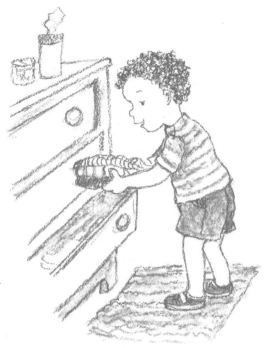

Another problem is the expectation of more and more that can come from giving gifts for ordinary good behavior. A child who becomes bored with simple, little gifts will expect more and more. By the time she is in fifth grade she'll be expecting a pony for making the honor role. Maybe that is an exaggeration, but overindulgence, even with young children, will only increase their reliance on material things. Like overeating, an unhealthy desire of material things can become a lifetime habit with unhappy results.

Be careful with your expectations of your children. Of course, responsible and caring parents want their children to do their very best, but we all have to be realistic. Not every child can graduate first in his class or be an Olympic athlete. It's wonderful to strive for the best, and with parental support and encouragement children can achieve a great deal. All children should grow up content and confident about their own personal gifts and talents. Pride in his or her accomplishments will help your child live a happy and productive life.

Parents shouldn't force a child to live out their own frustrated dreams of stardom. We have all been aware of adults who become overinvested in children's sports. A Little League coach may become enraged with his son for making an error. A high-achieving mother who hoped to skate in the Olympics may heap those unrealized dreams on her daughter. No matter what the circumstances, the children ultimately suffer in trying to achieve their parents' dreams.

Both criticism and praise must be handled carefully and gently with children. When given in an appropriate manner, constructive criticism can help children improve. When offered in an insulting and angry fashion, criticism can be hurtful and humiliating, sometimes with lifelong consequences.

On the other hand, praise has to be genuine, because even very young children will recognize when it is inappropriate and not heartfelt. Once again, it is a matter of courtesy and respect to show your child exactly what you yourself would hope to receive from others. Never be shy in expressing your love or in giving spontaneous hugs. True expressions of love will forge bonds that last a lifetime.

As Peggy has pointed out, children learn best by example, and there is no example more powerful in the lives of young children than their parents. Other caring adults, such as grandparents, aunts, uncles, family friends, and child care providers will make an impact on your child as well.

You are the most important role model in every instance.

This is why the example you set for your child is so critical. If you have older children, you will be helping them to become better parents themselves down the road by showing them how important it is to set a good example for their little brother or sister.

You can encourage good manners in a developmentally appropriate fashion from a very young age. Toddlers will initially just repeat "please" and "thank you" in a rote fashion when prompted, but will learn the true meaning of the words from your actions and example. Preschoolers are old enough to understand and even see for themselves how saying "please" and "thank you" in response to others' actions is a kind thing to do.

Children also learn by example with your tone of voice and manner and are quick to pick up the wrong words if they hear the adults around them using them. Very young children will pick up inappropriate words without knowing the meaning, but you can calmly and firmly explain that it is "not a word we use in this house." If they use a word in a more knowing fashion to prompt a response, make it clear that you are not pleased; what they want most is your attention and approval.

Good behavior can be reinforced by positive attention on your part. As Peggy and I continue to suggest, "Catch your child being good." You want to continue to heap praise on them consistently for good behavior and ignore the undesired behaviors. Children also need to see the adults around them behaving in an appropriate fashion in order to learn to do the same themselves. If you expect them to say "please" and "thank you" but never use the words yourself, they will be quick to sense the difference.

Honesty is also a part of good manners. Young children have an innate sense of justice and fairness and are quick to pick up on hypocrisy. If you insist your child wear his bicycle helmet, but he never sees you wear yours, what message are you giving him? Try to show your child good manners by example as well as by telling him what to do and what not to do.

Similarly, encourage your child to be true to his feelings. I always try to gently redirect parents who insist that a cowering child, who has just received a vaccination, give me a kiss goodbye in my office. That unhappy child most likely does not want to give me a kiss. Forcing a child to act

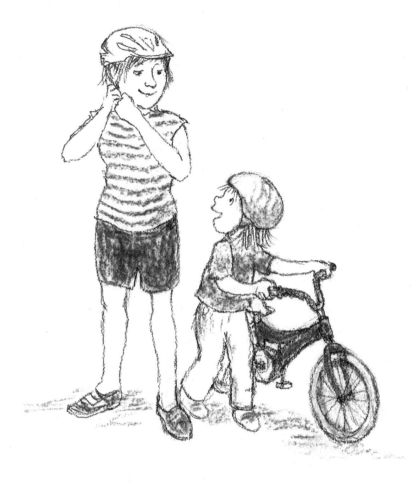

in a false fashion does not lay the groundwork for honest feelings and straightforward behavior later in life. Helping young children to express their feelings, both positive and negative, in a genuine fashion helps lay the groundwork for a lifetime of honest communication.

Asking your child to do small tasks around the house and then praising her for a job well done can also reinforce good manners. Children love to feel competent and needed, and even the youngest child can do simple tasks such as dusting, matching socks, and picking up her toys. Working side by side to accomplish a needed task in the house and then thanking her for her contribution helps a young child to see that her efforts are valued.

Your child will inevitably notice and comment on others around him who are not polite and do not use good manners. Watching people on a bus, seeing a television show, or noticing an interaction in the grocery store can be opportunities to discuss what is polite and what is not. Having these discussions in a discreet fashion, as opposed to the child pointing and making others around him uncomfortable, is also a learning opportunity.

As children get older it is always useful to help them learn that everything they see on television isn't necessarily true. Fostering critical skills will serve them well when they get to be older children and teens perusing sites on the Internet and again need to be reminded that everything they see there may not be true or accurate.

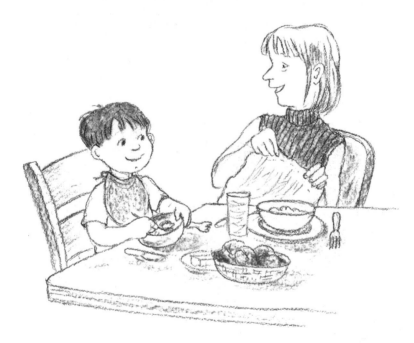

It is also important to have age-appropriate expectations of your child and her manners. Toddlers are not purposefully being rude when they have temper tantrums and start wailing. They are just overwhelmed by the situation at hand and need to be removed from the situation. A preschooler can be expected to understand and use please and thank you correctly but may be shy greeting new acquaintances and need reminders. Young school-age children can be expected to sit with adults at the table for a reasonable amount of time—say, 15 to 20 minutes—and be part of the conversation and mealtime interaction.

Helping your young children behave appropriately in different settings will help them cultivate lifelong skills for success in school and later in the workplace. There are many young adults entering the world of work who have impressive information technology skills but lack the social graces to function as skilled and polished team members. These young adults need to learn, often for the first time, the rudiments of social interaction such as introductions, shaking hands, and making a good first impression.

Among medical students I have the privilege to teach, those who are the most impressive are those who are already developing warm, compassionate communication skills to complement their growing and impressive funds of medical knowledge. I am confident they will become physicians who will be able to find the answers to their patients' solvable medical problems, as well as deliver the information compassionately when there are no easy solutions to those problems.

Finally, there is a part of good manners that is truly intuitive. We all know both children and adults who make us cringe and children and adults who are a joy and delight to be with. Pay attention to what you value most in the company of others. Then model and reinforce those traits for your own children. You will be helping them to develop the skills they need to develop into kind, polite, compassionate, and caring individuals.

CHAPTER 16

I Want a Puppy!

Pets and Children

A carefully chosen pet can become a beloved member of your family. It can be a good companion for your children as they grow up. For a child who is old enough to help care for a pet—whether that is walking the dog, feeding the cat, or cleaning the goldfish bowl—it can be a wonderful lesson in taking responsibility.

When our children were young, we always had pets. Even before they were born Dick gave me a parakeet, after he came home from the Korean War. We had only been married for six weeks before he was drafted. The gift of the parakeet came at the beginning of our married life together.

Later, when our children were small, we had a rabbit named Harvey, after the rabbit in the classic Jimmy Stewart film of the same name. Two cats lived with us in succession. Buffy, a big golden longhaired cat, came first, to be followed later by Ginger, a lively calico. When our son was eight, we were vacationing in Rockport, Massachusetts, on Cape Ann, and he announced that it would be a great idea for the family to get a dog. Although initially we only said we would consider the idea, choosing a dog became the children's summer project. They read every book they could find about dogs in the town's Carnegie library, researching which breed would be best suited to our family.

We all liked Airedales but decided that a smaller terrier would be better suited to life in the city. We decided to look for a Welsh terrier, which resembles the Airedale, only smaller. Later, we found a breeder in Connecticut, and Dylan Thomas the Welsh terrier became a beloved member of our family for the next seventeen years.

When our children were small, we lived with many generations of those little green turtles that you used to find near the cages of canaries and other birds, in the pet section toward the back of any Woolworth's store. Every autumn we were given beautiful goldfish from the pond outside of the Busch-Reisinger Museum, which housed Harvard's collection of Germanic art. The museum's caretaker was a friend who thought we would enjoy giving the goldfish a winter home.

Dylan was an excellent watchdog and would bark at any stranger arriving at our door. At the same time, he was wonderful with children, both our own and with my day care group. All the kids loved him. An eagerly anticipated event each year was Dylan's birthday party. I would make him a big hamburger "cake" with upright French fries substituting for candles. While the kids sang "Happy Birthday," Dylan would sit trembling, his tail thumping with excitement, as he waited for me to "blow out" the candles and serve him the hamburger.

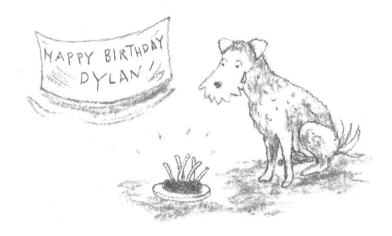

The children were wide-eyed with amazement as they watched Dylan gulp down his treat in several big bites. Then they would clap and cheer for the birthday dog, who was looking up at me as if to say, "Is that all?" With a pet, you're taking on the responsibility of caring for another living creature in your household, so be sure that you and your family have the time and patience to do so. Timing is everything, so make sure it is the right time in the life of your family to have an animal join your household.

While the right pet can be a wonderful addition to a family, the wrong choice can be a big disaster.

I knew of a man who gave his nine-year-old son a dog, shortly after the boy's mother died. A few weeks later he took the dog away, after the dog had been left alone all day in the house and made a mess. No doubt this father tried to do the right thing and just didn't foresee that in his situation a dog wasn't a suitable gift and didn't fit with their lifestyle. Maybe a goldfish or a bird would have been a better choice. For the child, the loss of the dog was yet another heartbreaking experience following the loss of his mother.

Introducing an existing pet to your new baby will require patience and understanding. Even though you will be busy with the baby, someone in the house or a friend who offers to help should try to give your pet the affection and attention it had grown accustomed to before the baby arrived. Never leave a baby alone with an animal. No matter how much you love and trust your dog or cat, be careful. Don't let your feelings blind you to the fact that your pet is, of course, an animal.

When properly introduced, a dog will soon accept the baby as part of the family pack and will even become protective of the child. A cat will probably continue to observe cautiously from an out-of-the-way perch. After adjusting, he or she is likely to adopt an unconcerned attitude and purr, as if to say, "Oh well, let's just live and let live."

When your baby begins to crawl, the problem will be reversed. You will constantly have to be on guard against the child hurting your pet. A pulled tail or ear will drive even the most docile dog or cat to respond with a snap or a scratch. Keep an eye out for children who may decide to share the food in Spot or Fluffy's dinner bowl. It is very important to teach your child how to be kind to your pet and how to make it happy by treating it gently and stroking its fur.

Once I cared for a one year old whose parents decided to add a large Belgian shepherd to their household in a city apartment. Understandably protective, they were terrified every time the dog and child went near each other.

Before giving up on the dog they consulted a renowned Boston canine psychologist about whom they had read in the *New York Times*.

After making several house calls, each for a considerable fee, to observe the interactions of the family with this dog, the psychologist concluded that there was nothing wrong with the dog or the child. It was the parents, who were too rigid and controlling. Gee, I could have told them that for nothing. Once the child's parents relaxed, the dog and the child got along well and the dog remained a part of the family for years.

Of course, a pet can be an added expense to the family budget. When we would go overseas for vacation, we would board Dylan out in Concord at a farm. The kids would try to prepare him by telling him he would have a good time on his vacation in the country. Believe me, Dylan was happy when we returned.

Dog care in my neighborhood is a good business. Dog walkers abound, and there is a local pet shop that also serves as a doggie "day care." Parents with dogs will sometimes walk with their dogs to drop off or pick up their children from my house.

Sadly, all things do end, and all pets have a relatively short life cycle or something untoward happens. My parakeet caught a cold. Our many turtles died, only to be replaced by identical new turtles so that the children wouldn't notice they weren't just sleeping inside their shells. Sometimes Dick would tell them it was time he took the turtles to the Charles River so they could swim away and grow big.

The loss of a beloved family pet is always very sad, yet at an appropriate age a pet's death provides an ideal opportunity to introduce children to the mystery and wonder of the life cycle. After our dog Dylan was euthanized, I told my day care group that he had gone to "doggie heaven," which sounded fine to them. After all, heaven sounded like a nice place.

Certainly a pet will be an additional responsibility, but if you choose wisely and pick a pet that fits your family's lifestyle it will give your children years of joy. Later, thoughts of the pet will be the basis for many happy childhood memories.

What a delightful image it is of Dylan, the Welsh terrier, gulping down his "birthday" cake surrounded by excited, adoring children. The perfect fit between family and pet can lead to many positive experiences and happy memories. It is important to think what type of pet suits your family best and how will you work out the logistics of caring for that animal over the course of its lifetime.

If you already have a pet when you bring your new baby home, you will have to introduce your cat or dog to the baby. Giving the animal a piece of clothing the baby has worn to sniff and become acquainted with the

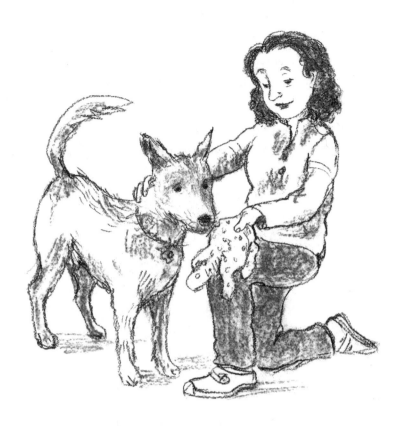

baby's smell is a good first step. After your pet has done so, with your careful supervision, let the animal into the same room as the baby.

Dogs will want to sniff the baby right away, while cats may watch from afar. When I brought my daughter home from the hospital, my cat Sophie jumped up on the bed, where Abby was sleeping quietly in a Moses basket. Sophie took one look, hissed, and hid under the bed. She took a while to readjust but quickly became a favorite of my children over the years. One of my daughter's first words was "cat."

When choosing a new pet for your house with small children, think about where your family may be in several years and imagine how that cat, dog, or rabbit will fit in. Dogs, in particular, need a lot of time and attention, and your busy family with small children might not be ready for that commitment. A dog can't be left alone all day, so you will need to arrange for "doggy day care" or a dog walker to visit if you are all away from the house for the entire day. Families with an in-home nanny or babysitter have sometimes arranged with that person to walk the dog as well as provide child care. Cats enjoy human companionship but are much more tolerant of being left alone for long stretches of time.

I learned firsthand about the importance of setting limits for dogs, as well as small children, when a friendly and very lively beagle named Louie joined our household a few years ago. Just as with parenting young children, training a dog requires a lot of patience and consistency from everyone involved. Good behavior needs to be constantly reinforced. Imagine my chagrin when during an important meeting at my home about this book, Louie grabbed a cookie right off the plate of our editor.

A small animal in a cage, such as a hamster, guinea pig, or gerbil can be a good pet for a preschool or school-age child, and its care is much simpler on a daily basis. Children have to be taught from the beginning how to handle the animal safely and gently to avoid scaring it. Small rodents will bite as a protective defense if handled roughly.

You also want to avoid bringing home an eagerly anticipated new pet to join your family only to realize that you have made a big mistake. The difficulty of finding a new home for the animal will be a chore, and the loss to your children can be quite upsetting. If you're not sure, spend more time researching on the Internet, visit local veterinarians and animal shelters to ask questions, and spend time as a family with friends who have pets before taking the next step of committing to a new animal.

Be sure to consider any health issues that might influence your choice of a pet. Children with asthma and allergies should avoid furry or feathered pets. Fish or a small reptile such as a chameleon would be better choices. Some breeds of dogs do wonderfully with children, while others regard them as intruders and look to attack. Just as Peggy's family did, be sure to research carefully your choice of a specific breed to find a dog whose personality suits a house full of children and whose activity needs can be met in the time you have available.

Pets in the household can occasionally transmit infection, so it's important to stress good hand washing after handling pets, cleaning cages, or picking up after their pets. Skin diseases can sometimes be transmitted from animals to people. *Tinea capitis*, or ringworm, is a skin fungus. Occasionally cats or dogs can have ringworm and pass it on to the people in their lives. If your children have recurrent ringworm it is a good idea to ask your veterinarian about skin testing any animals in the house.

Group A beta hemolytic streptoccal infections can be transmitted from dogs to humans, so be aware that your child could catch "strep throat" from the family pooch, as well as from another child. Reptiles can sometimes be carriers of the bacteria *Salmonella*, so be sure to mention that pet iguana to the pediatrician if your child has a persistent case of diarrhea. Thorough hand washing or use of an antibacterial hand sanitizer will prevent any of these problems.

Safety with pets as well as with other activities is essential. Pets should never be left alone with a baby or young child. Breeds of dogs bred to be guard dogs need to be taught very carefully about their small human family members, otherwise they may demonstrate aggressive behavior. It is also essential to teach young children never to pet unfamiliar animals without permission from the owner. Not all animals are friendly, and some will not be comfortable with the approach of an unknown young child.

Responsibility is a large part of owning a pet. Be sure that your expectations of what a child can actually do in caring for an animal are reasonable.

In the end, the care of that animal falls to the parents, with the children helping out. Very young children can fill food or water bowls; older children can clean cages, walk dogs, and even tidy up the cat litter box once they have been shown how to do so carefully. Getting home on time to walk the dog, or arranging for a neighbor to feed the cat all help show your children how important it is to meet your commitments and care for a living thing.

Pets are very helpful to children as they deal with feelings about certain issues or events. Talking over a problem with a sympathetic pet can be very therapeutic, and playing catch with a friendly active dog can make lots of worries disappear. A good-tempered, well-behaved dog or a friendly, affectionate cat can be a lot of company for an older child.

Dealing with issues of birth or death as they occur with the animals in your household also raises opportunities for discussion with your children. A litter of hamsters raises all sorts of interesting questions. Working through the sad feelings that accompany the death of a beloved cat or dog can help a child learn to understand death in a developmentally appropriate way. When the child later faces the death of a close family member they will be better equipped to know how to face the loss and actively cherish their memory when they are gone.

Pets are a great addition to a family, in a big way or a small way. Whether a tiny hermit crab in a terrarium, a huge friendly Bernese mountain dog, a regal Siamese cat, or any of the many other possibilities, children can learn an enormous amount about love, commitment, and responsibility. Choose a pet wisely, and choose one that suits your family, and you will be enhancing your family's experiences and creating lasting memories.

CHAPTER 17

Come Fly with Me!

Traveling with Children

Traveling with children can be fun. I don't necessarily mean you have to travel a great distance, although I will discuss vacation trips as well as short trips close to home. Just because you have a toddler doesn't mean you have to be a "stay-at-home" family. It's wonderful practice for children to take them out to restaurants, children's concerts, and plays. It teaches them how to act when they go out into the big world.

When our children were small, Saturday was always a big family outing, with exciting visits to the Museum of Comparative Zoology at Harvard, subway trips into Boston, where we would ride the famous Swan boats, or summertime trips by commuter rail up to Cape Ann. During these outings, we would take our time, adapting ourselves to the children's leisurely pace. We would always be sure to stop for a long lunch in a pleasant restaurant.

By the time we took our first long vacation journey, sailing from New York to Genoa on the Italian liner SS *Michelangelo*, our children were used to dining out, and the ship's grand dining room didn't faze them. Our son was four years old and our daughter was eight when we took that long voyage across the Atlantic into the Mediterranean Sea, with ports of call at Cannes and Naples.

A ship is a surprisingly child-friendly place. Many young families are reaching the same conclusion and travel on cruise ships that cater to travelers with children. On board, children can be looked after by the ship's trained staff when they want to be off playing away from their parents. I remember that our children seemed to love every second, splashing about in the ship's pools (there was a wading pool for tots), enjoying the toys in the well-stocked playroom, and joining us on deck for games of shuffleboard.

Dining with children in a ship's restaurant, or any other pleasant eatery for that matter, can be a delightful experience as long as they are well behaved. Our children had dined in restaurants many times before the voyage, so they knew just what was expected of them. During meals they would sit quietly at the table and were always polite to the wait staff. Of course, we didn't expect them to eat the elaborate multicourse meals we were offered. The good-natured Italian waiters, who took genuine delight in the children, would readily bring small portions of favorite foods such as pasta, tuna, cold cuts, and, of course, ice cream.

In Italy we traveled by train across the "boot" from Genoa to Venice, before going on to Florence and finally visiting my sister Egle, who lives in the Eternal City of Rome. August was hot, and most of the trains in those days weren't air-conditioned. Still, the children didn't fuss and would sit in the breeze of the open window, fascinated by the unfamiliar countryside and occasionally nodding off for a nap.

In each city we visited, the children walked about with us taking in the sights. When we grew tired we took some form of public transportation. In Venice a gondola ride was a must. We fed pigeons in St. Mark's Piazza, strolled through the Uffizi Gallery, and were awed by the grandeur of the Vatican. Having grown up in a small city, our children were used to walking everywhere and made good tourists. Like most children, they easily adapted to a different culture. While staying in Rome they were soon out in the street playing with all the children in my sister's neighborhood; the language barrier didn't seem to matter a bit.

We continued to travel with our children for many years—by ship, plane, and train—and it was always a joy. They were never a problem, because like the children in my day care, they were taught good manners in our home. During all our trips we made sure that the children had a midday nap or rest after lunch. There is no point in trying to do too much, because tired children will naturally be cranky and no one will have fun. After a good rest we would all be ready to go back out and explore.

Travel can certainly take many forms, whether short trips by city bus, a lengthy ocean cruise, or anything in between. I've told you about this particular trip with our children to illustrate the almost endless possibilities of travel with children. Properly prepared, they will enjoy the trip and all of you will share many happy memories. Don't hesitate to take them along; all too soon they will be going off on their own.

Good manners are always the key to good behavior. I don't approve of those "kiddie-friendly" restaurants where children are allowed to run about. A restaurant is not a playground, and children should learn the difference. I imagine it must seem like an easy night out for busy parents who might be reluctant to enforce appropriate behavior, but how will your children ever learn to behave in a "sit-down" restaurant if you never take them?

Over the years, I've often taken my day care group on day trips. Of course, for young children a short bus ride can seem like a thrilling journey. One time we took Boston's Red Line subway all the way to Braintree when a new line opened. We brought along bagels and juice for snacks and made a day of the trip.

Spotting our whole group of six children and me all sitting together in the train's first car, the motorman asked if one of the children would like to sit in the front with him to help "drive." Joey, the oldest child, seemed the most eager, so I allowed him to go. It's a thrill he still remembers as a young adult.

During the winter, weather permitting, we would take the bus and subway to Boston's Children's Museum for a day of indoor fun. In the

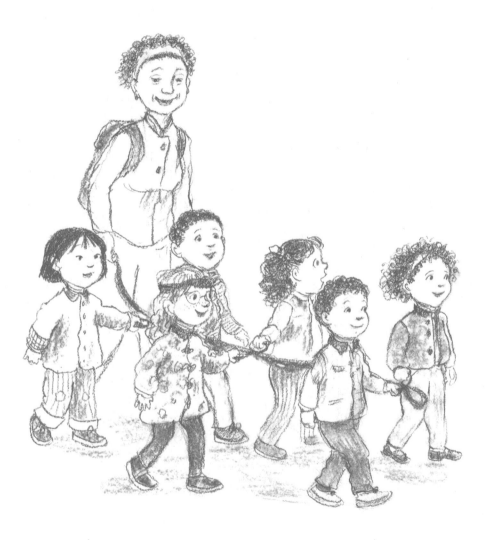

springtime we would often visit the Public Gardens in downtown Boston, the oldest public park in America. Here the children could sit on the bronze statues of the eight little ducklings by artist Nancy Schon, inspired by one of our favorite stories, *Make Way for Ducklings* by Robert McCloskey. They loved to look at the pond and imagine the eight ducklings and their parents happily paddling among the swan boats, being fed peanuts by the tourists.

We often just walk to the local park, always emphasizing that it is important to hold hands and never, ever run ahead. It really upsets me when I see children running ahead of their parents, out of control, on sidewalks next to busy city streets. Again, it is important for children to know the expectations of how they should behave in different situations. Most children readily respond to gently enforced limits set by the adults around them, but when parents never have any expectations of how their children should behave when out and about, they unwittingly create problems that can end up as nightmares for their own family and fellow travelers alike.

Certainly good manners are a must when flying in the close confines of an airplane, traveling by train or bus, or in the family car. Continue to encourage and enforce your "good-manners" rules, and fellow travelers will remark on how well behaved your children are. You will be proud, and enjoy the trip much more. With thoughtful preparation, gentle limits, and patience, family travel near and far can be enjoyable for everyone. So, take a trip, and make your own happy scrapbook of memories.

A love of travel with our families is something else Peggy and I share. My children were on their first planes within months of their births to visit our far away family, and we continue to enjoy travel in all forms. Children are natural explorers and love to learn about new places and people, whether a bus ride or a continent away. Day trips or long journeys all add to their experience and create treasured memories for your family.

All forms of transportation fascinate young children, so, as Peggy noted, a bus or subway ride can be a trip in itself. A bus ride to a new park on a sunny day can be a delightful way to spend time with young children, especially after reading stories about buses and singing favorite songs. For some children a bus or subway ride is part of their everyday experience in traveling to day care, so they will especially enjoy a leisurely walk to a nearby park on a weekend or holiday. As Peggy noted, cranky tired children are no fun to take anywhere, so making sure children are well rested and that you have plenty of time to get from one place to another is critical. Being flexible about what the experience provides is also helpful for children and adults alike.

Preparation and expectations are the key to successful travel with children, on any length trip, whether an everyday short trip to child care or a long journey to another country.

A trip to a museum with young children can be lots of fun. Museums have open corridors, lots of people, and innumerable wonderful things to look at. The adults do have to be prepared to look at all those things at a child's leisurely or rapid pace. Many museums now offer audio tours for children and children's activities on weekends and holidays. Museums often have free or reduced-price admission at certain times, and your local library may have passes to borrow.

Eating out with children can be an enriching experience for the whole family, especially if you plan ahead. Make sure your child can sit through a meal at home before trying it in a restaurant. Elaborate meals can be challenging for very young children, but a casual meal in a place that welcomes children is a treat for the whole family. Most restaurants are happy to be helpful, and you can often request a simple substitution such as pasta without sauce or a hamburger even if not on the menu.

Ordering an appetizer that comes out quickly for your child to start in on can save the meal. I can remember many meals in restaurants in which my children would happily eat their way through an order of French fries (something we rarely had at home) while waiting for the rest of the food to arrive. Pulling out a storybook or coloring book is always a good way to pass the time waiting for a meal to arrive. (This also works when waiting for a bus or a train.)

Some special notes about air travel with children are helpful. At this writing, children under the age of two can still sit on parents' laps without their own seat, but it is likely that will change in the future. The safest way for young children to travel by air is in their own car seats, buckled into their own adult seats, but that dramatically increases the cost for young families.

Be sure to let the airlines know you are traveling with a baby or small child, and even with reservations made on the Internet it is worth a special call to make the arrangements. Children's meals can also be requested if the flight is long enough that food is served, although food service is being phased out on many flights. Pack your own food for the children if food is not available on board. The front row in a cabin, or "bulkhead," seat provides a little extra room when traveling with small children and can be requested ahead of time.

Make sure babies are nursing, or have a bottle or a pacifier to suck, at the time of takeoff and landing to help them equalize the pressure in their ears. Flight attendants are willing to warm up bottles or baby food if you need it. Be sure to travel with a well-stocked diaper bag and plan for what you will need if you encounter travel delays. Older children can carry their own backpacks with books, toys, snacks, and a favorite toy or blanket to help the travel time pass.

A tricky time to travel is with a toddler who has just learned or is learning to walk. This is a child who does not want to stay in her seat. You and your fellow travelers will all enjoy the flight more if you arrive at the airport with plenty of time to let her run around and wear herself out before you board the plane.

Overseas travel to countries where the food and water safety is not assured requires a trip to the pediatrician beforehand. You can review any required travel vaccinations and discuss special precautions needed. If the water is not safe, remember to use only boiled or bottled water for drinking, cooking, and brushing teeth to avoid ingesting bacteria from the water. Watch out for ice cubes.

Fruits and vegetables should be peeled or cooked, not just washed, to avoid any bacteria that might cause travelers' diarrhea. Food from street vendors in countries where the water is not safe to drink should be avoided as well.

Remember to pack needed children's health essentials because searching for equivalent brands in a foreign country when your child has a fever can be nerve-wracking. I suggest families bring the following:

» Acetaminophen or ibuprofen for fever control and pain relief.

» Diphenhydramine (Benadryl) for allergy symptoms or itching.

» Sunscreen for children with an SPF (sun protection factor) of 30 or greater.

» Insect repellent for children (Deet concentration of 10 percent or less).

» Antibiotic ointment for scrapes, blisters, or burns.

» Moisturizer for dry skin.

» Thermometer.

» Assorted bandages, tape, and gauze.

» Packets of rehydration solution (Gerber LiquiLytes® or other brand).

These packets are easy to tuck into a suitcase. They can be mixed with boiled or bottled water to supply extra fluids to prevent dehydration in a baby or young child who gets diarrhea while traveling.

Traveling with a breastfed baby is easy and safe. If the baby is drinking formula, bring your favorite brand of powdered formula and mix it with boiled or bottled water. Bring along some of the baby's favorite cereal as well. For older children, pack some favorites such as granola bars or graham crackers to help ease the transition to new foods.

While traveling, you may find yourself in a strange city with a sick child. I have had calls and e-mails from around the world from my families who are traveling to interesting places. Check with your pediatrician before leaving on your trip, but most providers will be happy to have their staff give advice over the phone for simple problems while you are traveling. If you are uncertain about whether to take your child to the hospital in a foreign city, they can be helpful in pointing out what to look for and when to seek help, depending on what resources are available.

As Peggy noted with her own family, travel creates shared memories for the family. Whether a familiar bus ride, a short car ride to visit nearby family, or a long-awaited family vacation to far away, children love the anticipation and planning as well as the travel itself. Reading stories about where you are going, talking about what you will do at your destination, and then reliving the trip with photographs and scrap books—"Remember when we saw this?"—are delightful ways of enhancing your travel experience with your children. As one of our local travel agents is fond of saying, "Please, go away often!"

CHAPTER 18

Disasters

When Scary Things Happen in the World

It is unavoidable that children today will be exposed to the media. It is difficult, if not impossible, to shield them from the world's tragic events. Terrorist attacks, war, earthquakes, floods, and hurricanes are daily breaking news. Poignant television images of frightened families clinging to roofs during the aftermath of Hurricane Katrina prompted children all over the country to ask their parents, "Can that happen here?"

I comforted the children in my care when they asked about the flooding by saying that the flooding was far away and that they would be safe and snug in their own homes with their families. Usually the younger children in my care are more indifferent to current events. I did care for a four year old who began to have nightmares after the tragic events of September 11, 2001. He had seen several television news broadcasts of the hijacked jet planes crashing into the World Trade Center. This was a terrifying image for most adults, so it's no wonder the child had nightmares. Not only did he have nightmares, but he was also afraid to fly when his parents wanted to visit family. With some help from a child psychologist and the passage of time, the nightmares have resolved and the child now happily accompanies his parents on vacation flights.

I can recall the hurricane of 1938, which roared up the northeastern seaboard, causing massive destruction of property and nearly a thousand deaths. I still remember the torrential rains and howling winds snapping off tree branches on our street, but I don't remember being afraid. I was reassured that we were together as a family and felt safe. The next day the sun was shining brightly, and I went out with my brothers and sisters to join the other neighborhood kids playing on the street. We pretended we were in a jungle of broken branches and fallen trees and thought it was wonderful to have time off from school.

When my brothers went off to war after the attack on Pearl Harbor, I was twelve years old. Although I was very sad, the adults had helped us understand the necessity of their military service. As children we wanted to do our part for the war effort, so we collected scrap metal and newspapers for recycling and saved our pennies to buy War Bond stamps at school.

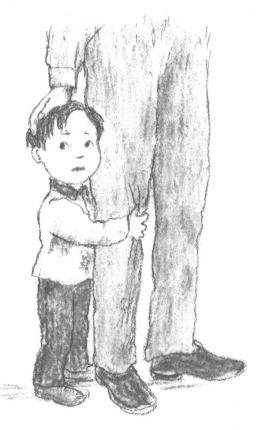

Beyond frequent air raid blackouts and the rationing of food and clothing, the war initially seemed far away. One day, though, a telegram came telling my sister that her husband was missing in action. He never came home again.

The first big world event my husband remembers is the plane crash that killed the famous cowboy entertainer Will Rogers. As the grownups were excitedly discussing the terrible crash in Alaska, Dick remembers wondering, "Where's Alaska?" Their answer that Alaska was a faraway place somewhere near the North Pole was enough to satisfy his curiosity. I find that with children you don't have to go into great detail when answering a question. What they ask is probably what they really want and need to know. As a young boy, Dick must have been more interested in Alaska than in what happened to Will Rogers.

I've read that watching too much television can be bad for children of any age, especially for those under the age of two. It can also be too stimulating for older children and very frightening. That wicked witch in the movie classic *The Wizard of Oz* can terrify even older children. Growing up in the days of radio dramas, I can still remember some very scary mystery programs. The famous Orson Welles radio broadcast of *The War of the Worlds* caused even adults to panic when they thought that Martians were actually landing in New Jersey.

Imagination is a wonderful gift, but, unchecked, it can run wild and be disturbing to children. When I was little, I was afraid of and used to hide from the "ragman," who went from door to door to collect old rags and sharpen knives. I suppose he was a harmless old man, just a bit disheveled. Children are most prone to fears and fantasies in the preschool years and will often be afraid of the dark. They will ask their parents to search for monsters under the bed or in the closet. A night light and reassurance can be helpful at this age.

During the Vietnam War, our neighborhood near Harvard University in Cambridge, Massachusetts, was often the scene of violent antiwar protests. Store windows were smashed, both in Harvard Square and at our neighborhood grocery store. State troopers carrying riot gear fought with the protesters, who had marched into Cambridge from Boston.

The sound of police and fire sirens could be heard often well into the night. Dick and I reassured our children that we would keep them safe from harm. These outbursts of violence began to seem almost routine, and the children just carried on with their normal activities.

During the blizzard of 1978, which virtually closed down New England, we were very fortunate. The storm, which completely shut down many communities in the greater Boston area for an entire week, was like a winter holiday for our family. People cross-country skied on the

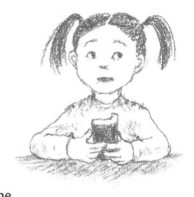

traffic-free streets and sledded across the frozen Charles River, but the storm was truly a disaster for many families whose homes were destroyed and whose loved ones were marooned in snowdrifts in their cars for hours. Families living near the shore had homes washed away by the surf generated by strong winds. One of my brothers and his family had to be rescued by the National Guard in an amphibious "duck" vehicle.

As a child care provider I always have a disaster plan in my mind just in case I have to hurry out of the house with the children. Years ago I lived on the second floor of a different house while providing child care. A careless workman on the first floor caused an explosion when a lit cigarette ignited a flammable substance on the floor. Black smoke streamed up through the heating vent into our apartment. I quickly picked up the baby, and gathered up the three preschool age children I was also caring for at the time. I calmly told them to start walking down the stairs and that I was right behind them. There was no panic, and within seconds we were sitting on the steps of the house next door. The children loved all the activity as firefighters, police, and many onlookers arrived at the scene. Despite the billowing smoke, it was just a small fire. Fortunately no one was badly hurt, and the poor workman received only some minor burns. Other than some smoke damage in the kitchen and a bedroom, our apartment was fine.

In another incident, a child I once cared for was rushed to the hospital for emergency treatment because her parent had left adult medication within reach at his home. Never imagine that a climbing child can't reach your medicine cabinet. Some small children will taste anything; I know a child who licked a paintbrush she found soaking in a can of paint thinner in her house. Fortunately all the children I have cared for have been fine after their accidents, with appropriate medical attention.

Of course, it isn't possible to be prepared for every conceivable natural disaster, which can strike at any time. Careful parents can do many things to help prevent the human-driven disasters closer to home, such as kidnapping or child molestation. We instructed our children years ago—and I do the same with my child care group—not to talk to strangers who might stop them on the street.

We tried to strike a reasonable balance between careful fear and caution. We told our children that it was okay to speak to "safe grownups" such as a police officer, the parents of their friends, teachers, or any mother of small children. These were the people they should go to if they needed help.

With small children, it is so important to maintain the safety of your house and to be vigilant about accident prevention at all times.

When caring for children you must always think of safety first, and never take anything for granted. We can't prevent big storms or acts of terrorism, but our children will be safer if we prevent the small household disasters and have a plan in response to the big disasters.

We live in a complex world. As parents of young children, we want to protect them as much as possible from the darker side of this complexity. Even if you shield your child as much as possible from the media, you will find its influence to be pervasive. Apparently my daughter kept a close eye on the O.J. Simpson trial back in the 1990's. During naptime, when the children were all supposed to be sleeping, Peggy would occasionally turn on the television for a news update. Abby was vigilant about staying awake as she knew it must be something important if the grownups were so interested.

The impact of television and the graphic images often presented are more reasons to be careful with young children's television time. Under no circumstances should the television simply be left on as background sound and images. When children see complicated images and become afraid of what they have seen, it is very important for the adults around them to sit down, watch for a few moments with them, and explain in very simple terms what they are seeing. As Peggy has noted, a simple explanation answering just what the child has asked is best.

Terrorist attacks and the unthinkable violence and havoc wreaked have become an unwelcome reality here in the United States and have been a part of the daily reality in other parts of the world such as the Middle East for much longer. Children will want to know why some people will choose to detonate bombs and hurt others, including those they do not know. It is useful to come up with a simple answer that can be repeated because children will often ask over and over again. You might simply say, "Sometimes people do very dangerous things, for reasons we just can't understand."

Much has been learned about how children handle massive disaster in the aftermath of September 11, 2001. Children who were given an op-

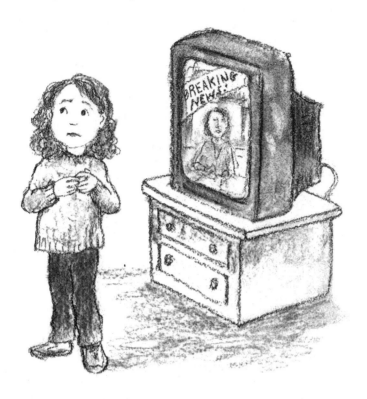

portunity to share and express their feelings did better overall and could move on more quickly. Art therapy was very useful to many children, and the drawings of young survivors are poignant and powerful. Children also did best when their surviving parents and caregivers helped them keep to their usual routine and made as few changes as possible in the early days following the tragedy. Mental health support is essential for both children and adults.

Children also need to know when worried about hurricanes or terrorists or any other larger-than-life events that their parents and other adults around them are doing everything they can to keep them safe. This is definitely a time for adults to keep their fears to themselves and not share them with children. Your children do not need to share your fears; they just need to know that you are doing everything necessary to keep them safe.

Limit your child's television viewing when hurricanes, blizzards, or other natural disasters are impending. Television networks do their best to inform the public but are also hoping for good ratings, and some are quite sensational in this sort of coverage. If children are sent home from school or child care because of an impending storm, seeing their parents calmly going about securing everything and making the necessary preparations will be very reassuring.

Once the storm logistics are seen to, use the time for games, stories, and other fun activities to make the time pass quickly and help dissipate any worries. Of course, if the situation is serious enough for your family to be evacuated, do your best to stay calm for your children. Pack the few things that will give them the most comfort, if you are to be in a shelter or other safe place away from home. In terms of the comfort it will give your child, a favorite stuffed animal, small picture album or story book, and a treasured quilt or pillow will be well worth the effort it takes to carry it. Remember to bring your child's birth certificate or passport and immunization record.

We want to help our children grow up strong and confident as well as friendly and outgoing with others. However, you also want to teach your children to have a reasonable degree of caution with strangers to keep them safe. Children should be taught to never take anything from strangers and never go off with strangers. Adults who prey on young children can be quite clever about telling children they are acting on behalf of a parent or teacher to win their confidence. It is useful to talk through some scenarios with your children at different ages, so they know how to say "no" and mean it in one of these difficult situations.

Through all disasters big and small in the lives of young children it is very important to stick to the child's routine. Children use familiar routines to make sense of the world and predict what comes next. When they sense that world is changing, it is very reassuring to them to be put to bed with the same bedtime routine, even if in a different place. Favorite foods, toys, and stories are also comforting. Stories about young children facing adversity are especially reassuring and empowering.

As parents, we strive to protect our children. It is a fact of life that we won't be able to prevent challenging events and natural disasters from occurring in their lives. Our task is to support them in every way possible and give them the tools to face whatever challenges life presents them; bravely, with humor, with love and with confidence.

CHAPTER 19

Fun and Games

Encouraging Imaginative Play

Don't we all remember our favorite toys and childhood games? When I was a little girl, as one of the youngest children in a large family, my toys were simple and inexpensive. A box of crayons, a bag of marbles, jacks, and a set of Pick-Up Sticks were among my childhood treasures. We used to make our own coloring books from cards with line drawings of classic children's stories that came in cereal boxes.

A piece of chalk was special. It could be shared with playmates for drawing the design on the sidewalk for our hopscotch games. Jump rope was fun; it's hard to believe now that I'm a senior citizen, but I could even jump rope Double Dutch style with two ropes at one time. I remember lots of the jingles we used to sing, including one that ended with all the kids shouting "23 Skidoo!" as we tossed our jump ropes aside.

On hot summer evenings the parents in the neighborhood would sit out on their front stoops and watch the children play. Sometimes the boys would let me bat because I was a good left-handed hitter. I usually played hide and seek with the girls and younger boys, until the game ended in the fading twilight. The kid who was "It" shouted, "Allee allee in free!" as the parents called us in for bedtime.

A highlight every spring was the May Day parade of toys held in the playground of our local park. All the neighborhood children would make colorful costumes and decorate their doll carriages, wagons, and tricycles with the crepe paper the playground supervisor handed out. Some of our children's favorite toys were also the simplest: blocks, Lincoln Logs, stuffed animals, Tonka trucks, and a dollhouse. These toys, along with lots and lots of books, freed their imaginations for many hours of creative play.

Even now in this high-tech age the children in my care love to play with these types of toys. In my living room I have a stack of five plastic storage boxes, each a different color and each full of different types of toys. After the children arrive in the morning, I read a story and then let them choose what they want to play with.

Among the toys are alphabet and Lego blocks, a boat, a yellow school bus, a wooden mailbox, and a dollhouse with tiny figures of a family. While playing with these toys the children invent their own stories, building castles and trains or taking the little family for a boat ride out to sea, across the living room rug.

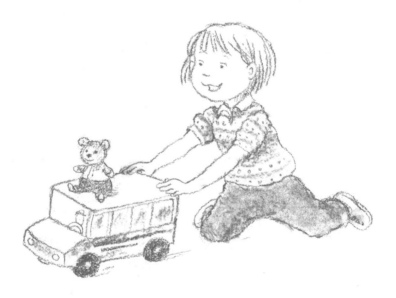

We also have lots of picture books, puzzles, and flash cards of letters and shapes that I use to play educational games. I always emphasize fun and don't believe in creating a stressful day for the children. In the afternoon we often sing songs together. They quickly learn the words to "The Wheels on the Bus," "Here We Go 'Round the Mulberry Bush," and "Hush Little Baby." If I make a mistake in the words, they are quick to call out, "That's wrong, Peggy!"

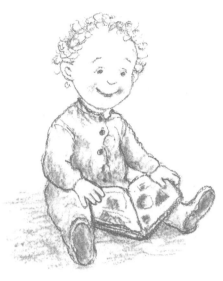

The television is rarely on in my house. Occasionally we will watch a favorite short video or a half hour of children's programming. I worry that children today watch too much television and don't have enough opportunities to imagine the stories they've been read.

Growing up before television, on rainy afternoons I listened to the radio serial dramas *Orphan Annie* and *Jack Armstrong*. Listening to the radio is a lot like being read to by a grownup. We had to visualize every scene in our imaginations. Now children expect to see everything on television. I recently played an audio recording of the music from the movie *The Wizard of Oz* on my old record player. The children ran over to the television, and were stunned when they looked at the blank screen. Concerned, they ran back to me, asking, "What's the matter, Peggy?"

Along with teaching the children good manners and setting limits I want them to enjoy their day together. I remember the years of unstructured play my siblings and I enjoyed as children, before entering school at the now-advanced age of five. Today children seem to have fewer opportunities for this kind of play, often entering fairly structured preschools at the age of three. I've even known parents who have approached the preschool admission process with the same intensity as if the child was applying to an Ivy League college. If the child is rejected, the parents fall into a prolonged period of depression. Fortunately most children remain oblivious of the disaster and happily carry on, unaware of the enormity of this failure at the ripe old age of three.

It's too bad, because it seems to me that's a lot of unnecessary pressure to put on a child as well as the parents, and, frankly, it seems silly. I never put any stress on the children in my care and the parents are always satisfied with what I teach them. They often come back to tell me that their preschool asked them where their child had gone to child care because the school was impressed with the child's good manners and behavior.

I wonder what toys these children from my child care group today will remember when they are grownups? Children are children, and I imagine it will be something simple like a doll, stuffed toy, red wagon, set of blocks, or other favorite. Good toys rarely wear out and certainly never go out of fashion.

Good toys are magical. My son Andy, like my brothers when I was growing up, played for hours building structures with his Legos. My daughter had a treasured stuffed cat that went everywhere with her from the age of one. Being an animal lover, I played with a tiny mouse and her rabbit friend in a little cabin instead of a dollhouse. My mother saved the mouse house and many of our other treasured toys, which were then enjoyed by all her grandchildren.

Good toys are timeless, as Peggy has noted. The first toys were tiny dolls and animal figures carved out of stone or wood or made out of plant material. Board games with small pieces and a playing board or area marked out in the dirt date back to very early civilizations. Mancala, a counting game of skill with small marbles, pebbles, or other markers, was known to have been played in ancient Egypt in 1400 BC and is still played around the world in many different cultures and countries.

More recently, Candyland, a board game still popular with early school-age children, was invented in 1949. The graphics on the game board have been updated, but the essentials of the game are still the same today. Hasbro introduced Mr. Potato Head, a clever plastic potato with many interchangeable facial features and accessories, in 1952. Play-Doh was invented in 1956 and recently celebrated its fiftieth birthday. These are toys that have stood the test of time and remain popular with children today. They are simple, sturdy, and imaginative.

The key to good toys is choosing the right toys for your child's age. At each stage, look for toys that foster multiple experiences and allow for many responses. Toys that encourage problem-solving skills, such as games and puzzles, are also good for entertaining challenges.

Simple toys that can be used in different ways foster imaginative play for children of all ages.

Babies enjoy brightly colored rattles. I'm less fond of toys for young children with recorded or electronic sounds that play when pushed or poked because they only do one thing repeatedly. Activity sets or gyms with lots of brightly colored toys that hang down and can be batted around are fun.

Helping your child find a transitional object, a stuffed toy or blanket that is her special item to fall asleep with, is an important task. Some children never pick a transitional object, but most do. Something relatively

small, easy to cuddle, and hopefully
easy for you to wash will do the trick.
I've even known parents to buy dupli-
cates so that when the beloved stuffed
animal or blanky is being washed
there is something to take its place.

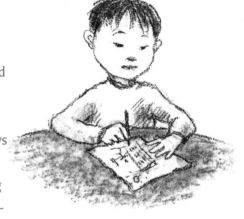

Toddlers start to enjoy building toys
like blocks and big Legos. Toys that
involve sorting, stacking, and putting
smaller pieces into compartments be-
gin to fascinate children at this age. They begin to play with toys actively,
banging and making cars go. Dolls and animals are moved around actively
and carried with them many places.

This is also the age when children love to empty out cabinets, bang
spoons, and play with nesting plastic containers. Your kitchen is a wealth
of potential toys, and having a cabinet that children can explore and
empty can keep them busy while you work in the kitchen as well.

Preschoolers begin to be very engaged in stories and imaginative
play. Not long ago I watched a four-year-old child at Peggy's engaged in
an elaborate play story with the dollhouse and tiny figures of the family
members. The child was speaking to herself and narrating an intricate
story of what was happening in the family's life.

Generic toys—ones that are not associated with children's television
characters or other media figures—foster more creativity and interaction.
Children may feel compelled to act out the specific plot of the movie or
television show the characters came from instead of engaging in a more
open-ended or creative form of play. A set of people or animals not tied to
any show or product affords more possibilities to children and encourages
more imaginative play.

It's never too early to start to avoid toys and other items that are merchandising and advertising for media ventures. It will only get worse when your child grows older and advertisers start promoting products directly to your child. Children can become obsessed with having a particular toy that is heavily advertised and the focus on acquisition of more material things takes the place of enjoying playtime.

When choosing toys, look for the following:

» No sharp or jagged edges.

» Nontoxic finishes.

» To avoid choking, no pieces less than 1.75 inches in diameter for children under three.

» Easy-to-find replacement parts.

» Expandable sets you can add to (especially with building sets).

» Durability.

» No projectile pieces.

It is wise to limit the number of toys your child has at one time. Too many are overwhelming, and your house turns into a toy store. You can even take some of the many toys your child gets for gifts and set some aside to bring out later. If you have extras, family shelters or local nonprofit child care centers can always put them to good use. Rotating the toys keeps things very interesting for your child and cuts down on the clutter. Sometimes family members

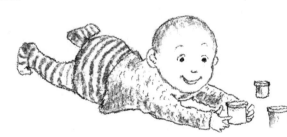

are delighted to contribute to your college fund instead of purchasing more toys.

Bribing children for good behavior with the promise of a new toy sends the wrong message. You don't want your children to expect that they will get something new each time they behave appropriately. Children need to learn to behave well because they want to and because they see you behaving that way. Good behavior is its own reward. They learn that life goes much more smoothly when everyone behaves well and treats each other with courtesy and kindness.

Watching children play creatively is a true delight. Often they will mix and match toys from different sets and origins to create their own new game or story. A doll can enjoy a ride around in a Tonka truck, and a stuffed animal can be dressed in doll's clothes. Legos are great for building barns and dollhouses as well as the more traditional buildings and bridges. An empty box can offer hours of fun as a fort, a house, a cave, or another imaginative possibility.

Play is the primary task of young children, and good toys will help children to play well. Toys are a good analogy for the rest of life. You and your child will find that the simpler and less complicated toys are often the best. Choose well, and your child will enjoy those toys for a long time.

CHAPTER 20

Read Me a Story

Fostering a Love of Reading

My day care children love when I tell or read them a story. They laugh out loud when I act out my own version of *The Three Little Pigs* and, as the Big Bad Wolf, "huff and puff" and can't blow the brick house in. Sometimes I do edit some of those old favorites to make the stories less violent and scary for the little ones.

I usually read to the children in the morning, after they settle down, and again after nap time. When I finish reading or acting out a story, I talk to the children about the plot to be sure they understand. One little girl comes to my house at midday from nursery school. The first thing Natasha does is to go to the bookcase to pick out a story for me to read to her, before she has lunch. One of her favorites is Hardie Gramatky's 1939 story *Little Toot on the Thames*, the story of a tugboat. After many adventures on the river in London, the tug comes back to America pulled by the old luxury liner SS *Queen Elizabeth*. As I read the story, she likes to tell me what comes next. "Here comes the queen!" she says before I turn the page and we see a picture of the ship.

I remember how much as a little girl I enjoyed the stories our teachers would read in school, such as *Rumpelstiltskin* and the *Little Shoemaker*. Story time was an eagerly anticipated treat. When we were older, we would take turns reading books such as *Black Beauty* aloud in class, one chapter at a time.

Because of our family circumstances, the younger children in my family didn't have anyone to read to us at bedtime. I do remember, though, that we had a Christmas Eve tradition involving a beloved story. My older sister Irene would bring out a battered copy of *The Night before Christmas* by Clement C. Moore and read to us as we sat together in the parlor.

My husband Dick says that his mother always read to him before he went to sleep. He recalls that his favorite books were Rudyard Kipling's *Just So Stories* and the *Snip, Snap, and Snurr* series by Maj Lindman. We both used to read to our children, taking turns at bedtime. I was home during the day when our children were young and would read to Wendy and Doug whenever they asked for a story. Among their favorite bedtime stories were *Little Bear* by Elsa Homelund Minarik and *Winnie-the-Pooh* by A. A. Milne.

Over the years I have found most of the children in my day care have loved books. I know that their parents enjoy reading to them at home as well. One of my "alums," Emily, came to visit me the other day and talked about her high school summer reading list. From a list of 100 books she chose ten to read over vacation. She said she looked forward to the assignment because there were a number of books she wanted to read but just didn't have the time. She tells me that she'll always remember the many stories I read to her during our years together. It's hard to believe, but she says she has nearly 400 books in her personal library. Emily is fortunate to have grown up in a home where reading has been encouraged and books are treasured.

I know several children whose family didn't have many books at home but who loved going to the library. The children I care for are taken to the library by their parents, often twice a week. Even our small branch library has a story hour. It's important for children to enjoy reading because it is a joy they will have for a lifetime. We were lucky that when our children were little the public library was right across the street in the middle of a park. Going to play in the park and then stopping at the library was a frequent routine.

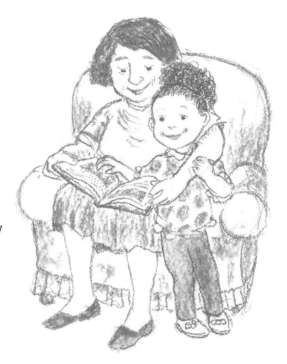

Growing up in Hartford, Connecticut, Dick says that his public library was located in Mark Twain's house. As a child, my favorite library was in nearby Somerville. Wherever we vacationed as a family we visited new libraries. Our children remember sitting in the town library in Rockport, Massachusetts, on lazy summer afternoons after a morning swim at the beach, with the hum of big fans in the background as they eagerly read new books.

The children in my day care haven't learned to read yet, but they love to look at the illustrations in my collection of children's books. Some of these books are more than forty years old and have been enjoyed by several generations—they're like old friends. The books are in good condition, because I teach the children to respect and treasure books.

We don't watch much television other than an occasional requested video or half hour of children's programming on our local PBS station. Because the television is rarely on, the children don't miss it. They would rather play with blocks, the dollhouse, and other toys or look at picture books themselves until I read them a favorite story.

Reading together is the single most important thing that you, as a parent, can do to prepare your child to succeed in school. But reading aloud to a child, as Peggy has reminded us, is more than a daily task to accomplish. It is a shared adventure, a time of closeness, and, most important, an enjoyable moment together during a busy day when parents and young children often spend lots of time apart.

Choosing the right book for the developmental stage of your child is essential. Very young children don't have the patience or concentration needed to sit through long intricate stories with complicated pictures and plots. Babies enjoy looking at black and white shapes on pages, as in the *Black on White* board books by Tana Hoban.

Older babies and toddlers love to look at books with bright faces of babies and toddlers, such as the *Baby Faces* board book series by Roberta Grobel. Helen Oxenbury has written and illustrated a number of simple, joyous board books in the *Big Board Book* series with titles such as *Tickle, Tickle* and *Say Goodnight*. These are favorites of mine and most babies. Both series show a variety of children from diverse ethnicities and backgrounds.

Preschool age children begin to have the patience and attention to enjoy longer stories. The field of children's literature has blossomed, and your children can enjoy classics from your childhood as well as new titles you find together. *Make Way for Ducklings*, written by Robert McCloskey in 1941, is set in Boston's Public Gardens. *Mike Mulligan and His Steam Shovel*, written by Virginia Lee Burton in 1939, still engages children to the last page.

Choosing from the thousands of children's books available is daunting. Since 1938 the Association for Library Service to Children (a division of the American Library Association) has awarded the Caldecott Medal annually to the artist of a notable picture book. Randolph Caldecott was a nineteenth-century illustrator in Great Britain, and the artists awarded the medal in his honor have created extraordinary illustrations.

Since 1922 the same organization has also presented the Newberry Medal to the author of the year's most notable book for children. John Newberry was a bookseller in Great Britain in the eighteenth century, and these are books for all ages of children with remarkable plots and superb writing. You can be sure of picking an extremely high-quality children's book if it is a Newberry or Caldecott Medal winner or one of the books listed on each award's annual honor list.

The books in the *Frances* series, about a badger and her family, by Russell Hoban and, except for the first one, illustrated by Lillian Hoban, were written more than thirty years ago and still are very useful for helping children work through conflicts. Read *Bread and Jam for Frances* to picky eaters and *A Baby Sister for Frances* when a new sibling is on the way.

Newer titles appropriate for three or five year olds depict children in a variety of settings and with different family groupings. *A Chair for My Mother*, by Vera B. Williams, centers on a little girl and her mother in an urban setting. *Everybody Cooks Rice*, by Norah Dooley, is a delightful book, complete with recipes, showing neighbors from different parts of the world preparing rice in different ways. The many beautifully illustrated children's books by Eric Carle with their lush colors and collages may inspire your own little artists.

As children get ready for kindergarten and first grade and approach the age when they will learn to read by themselves, they will often "practice" reading by memorizing the simple text of a picture book and reciting it by heart. This is wonderful because it is the beginning of actual reading and something you should encourage. The many Dr. Seuss books are perfect for this with their infectious rhymes and carefully limited vocabulary.

As Peggy has noted, taking your child to the library for story hour and to check out books can be a fun outing and builds the foundation for a life-long love of reading. Many libraries now have programming on Saturdays and in the early evenings to accommodate working parents. Bookstores also have children's story and activity hours and are a fun way to learn about new books and maybe even meet the authors.

There is a large body of current research confirming the positive effects of reading. Pediatricians are eager to share that information and encourage families to read. Reach Out and Read (ROR) is a visionary program started at Boston Medical Center in 1989 when pediatricians noted that books kept disappearing from the clinic waiting rooms.

The program has grown over the years to provide a framework for pediatricians and nurse practitioners to give children a new, developmentally appropriate book at each well child visit from age six months to five years. Along with the book to take home, parents and caregivers are coached about early literacy milestones and see volunteers reading in waiting rooms, modeling the desired interactions. If your doctor's office does not participate, ask someone to find out more and become involved.

Reading Is Fundamental (RIF) is another wonderful program that has helped foster a love of reading in generations of children since 1966. Now more than forty years old, the program supplies books to children in a variety of settings: child care centers, preschools, schools, and after-school programs as well as clinics and hospital-based programs. It is based on the key premise that all children should be able to choose the specific book they truly want to read. Even reluctant readers will enjoy reading or being read to when they have chosen the book themselves. Children can sit next to you for a moment and pretend to read the newspaper or a magazine.

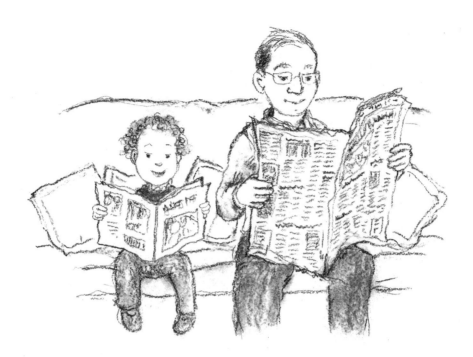

Parents can tell children how much they look forward to going to bed and reading, even if just for a few minutes at the end of a long day. Seeing a parent read on the beach or on a blanket in the park is a powerful model for young children. If your children see you reading, they will want to read as well.

As with so many other behaviors, your children will be more likely to love books if there are books in your house and they see you reading.

The reverse is also true. As Peggy reminded us, if you do not watch much television, neither will your children. The American Academy of Pediatrics has suggested that parents limit television very deliberately in their recent policy statement in 2001. Older children should watch no more than one or two hours of television every day. For children younger than two, television should be discouraged. We are just beginning to understand that the kind of stimuli television provides to the young brain of an infant is not healthy. Talking to a child, singing to them, reading to them, or engaging them in active play is all much better.

We know that television is very stimulating and should not be used as a babysitter or a bedtime sleep aid. More than a third of children from two through seven have televisions in their bedrooms. When parents are concerned about their child's sleep, one of the first questions I ask is "What about TV?" I try to emphasize to parents and children of all ages that a little television is all right, but a lot is most definitely not. For older children, don't forget to limit their total "screen time"; that is the cumulative amount of time spent in front of any screen: television, computer, and electronic games.

Finally, watching television is a solitary pursuit and not conducive to human interaction or connection. Reading aloud offers so much more. The warmth of a wiggly preschooler sitting on your lap, eagerly anticipating the next page, is a delightful interaction that can be one of the best parts of both of your days. Read to your children and you will both benefit immeasurably.

CHAPTER 21

To Grandmother's House We Go

Grandparents and Children

My grandson lives in a tiny country village in East Sussex, England. Teddy has lots of land to run around on, and when he gets older he can pretend he's a medieval knight. Herstmonceux Castle is just down the road from his parents' 400-year-old home. We visit at Christmas and look forward to visiting and playing with him every summer.

That's the wonderful thing about being a grandparent. You get to have all the fun of being with children without the daily responsibilities of parenthood. Of course, in some families grandparents take on partial or complete responsibility for the children. After his mother died, Dick lived with his grandmother until his father remarried.

In some families, grandparents are willing to provide full- or part-time care for their grandchildren. When everyone agrees on the details, this may be the best arrangement imaginable for young children and their parents. The only problem I can foresee is when conflict arises between parents and grandparents over how to handle problems. "In my day we did things this way" will likely lead to everyone putting their defenses up instead of thinking together about what is best for the child.

In the many years I've provided child care, I've enjoyed getting to know the grandparents of many of the children I've cared for. From time to time they've complained to me about how their children parent their grandchildren. Sometimes grandparents feel parents are too lenient, sometimes too strict, and often they do not feel their comments are welcome by the parents. I encourage them to offer advice only when asked, as I do with my own son and his wife in matters concerning my grandchildren. Grandparents can be a wonderful source of information on parenting and have a perspective developed over years of both parenting and grandparenting.

The older generation strikes me as more flexible in its attitudes now than was the case years ago. Grandparents are a wonderful source of family memories. Hardly a week goes by when Dick doesn't mention his grandparents and his boyhood summers in Vermont or his grandmother who cared for him when he was young.

Our grandmother in Italy raised one of my older sisters after my parents and sister Eleanor emigrated to America in 1920. Just before my family was to sail from Naples on the SS *Duca degli Abruzzi*, my sister Egle came down with measles and stayed behind with her beloved "nonna." She grew up in Italy, and it wasn't until 1967, when our family visited Rome, that Egle met anyone from the rest of her family.

This was often the case for new immigrants. Before travel was relatively inexpensive and available to all, many children would never know their grandparents left behind in "the old country." For many families, grandparents were only known as the people dressed up in old-fashioned clothes in photographs on the parlor mantelpiece.

Family stories are so important to children. When children understand their family's roots they can better understand their place in the world. Perhaps an ancestor fought in the Civil War, family members came to America on an immigrant steamer or slave transport ship, or ancestors escaped from the Holocaust. Family tales are an important part of our oral tradition and tie us to historical events. Even with the embellishments over the years—such as the modest house left behind in Naples now

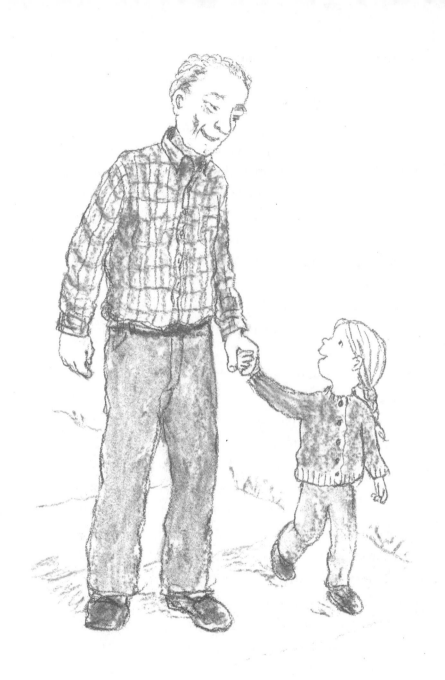

referred to as a villa or the grandfather who was a ship's steward and over the years is transformed into a captain—these stories become a rich part of every family's history.

All of the children in my care now are fortunate to have grandparents as a vital part of their lives. A four year old I care for went to Russia with his parents to visit his grandparents. Two girls in my group have visited grandparents in Minnesota and New York. A sibling pair sometimes stays with their "Baba" in New Jersey. We look forward to visits whenever possible with our grandchildren and their parents. They send cards to their "nonna" and granddad on Mother's Day and Father's Day, and we are overjoyed.

Whether down the block or across a continent, grandparents have a very special role to play in a child's life. Most grandparents have the delightful role of supplying unlimited amounts of unconditional love to their grandchildren. They don't have to worry about day-to-day responsibilities. They often are at a less complicated phase of their lives, with time and patience to spare for their grandchildren.

Grandparents are also able to be much more flexible and relaxed with children. In the best of circumstances at this later stage of life they are more secure and less likely to need to live out their dreams through their children and grandchildren. This allows them to more genuinely follow the child's lead and be truly present with them in the moment without the many pressures of busy lives felt by parents.

Grandparents can play an important role in their grandchildren's lives, no matter where they live. Those who live close by are fortunate to be able to visit frequently and share in daily activities, birthdays, school events, and other milestones. When grandparents live far away, letters, e-mails, and phone calls can maintain the connection to play an important role in their grandchildren's lives. One innovative grandmother reads to her grandchildren over the phone while the children hold the same book and turn the pages as they listen.

My children, niece, and nephew were always delighted to receive a package at every holiday with carefully chosen stickers, silly cards, and a cheerful note from their "Gramma Sara," my mother. She helped them learn to cherish the holidays and truly celebrate every day regardless of whether it was a holiday. Even though she lived two thousand miles away from her grandchildren, she played a vital part in their lives and visited whenever possible. We are all especially grateful for these memories now that she is gone.

During the busy lives of young families, there will be times when parents and grandparents disagree. How these situations are handled will vary from family to family. I agree with Peggy that it's a good idea for grandparents not to offer advice unless asked. One approach might be for grandparents to model different approaches to common problems when visiting.

For example, rather than engaging in control struggles with young children about eating, grandparents can demonstrate a relaxed way of sitting and eating with them and in the process cajole them to eat more. Instead of parents controlling and scheduling their activities, grandparents may have the patience to demonstrate open-ended imaginative play such as playing in the park or digging and planting in the garden. Parents may be surprised to see how well their children respond to these different approaches.

It is often helpful for parents and grandparents to acknowledge how different their lives may be. Grandparents may not have had the busy lives and schedules of today's parents, but may have had more pressures of war, unmet health needs, and financial shortfalls. Many of today's parents might have a higher standard of living, but they also have more hectic commutes and the stresses of two busy jobs or professions to contend with. These differences affect the lives of young children, and a frank discussion can clear the air and help ease any misunderstandings.

Sometimes the best that grandparents can do for their children and grandchildren is to acknowledge that life *is* complicated today and offer support in any way they can to help make the young family's life simpler. For example, a grandparent's offers to watch the grandchildren while parents run errands, or even have a night out for grown-up time, is lovely and supportive. Grandparents far away might offer to time their visit when the day care center or child care provider takes an annual vacation, so they can provide substitute child care.

It is important to note that some grandparents become the primary caretakers of their grandchildren, often under challenging circumstances. Their role is then much more like that of parents, with all the daily responsibilities of caring for those children. They have the benefits of their age, wisdom, and patience and the disadvantages of any of their own age-related health or other issues. They may also have their own losses to struggle with, such as the untimely death of their own child that has brought about the need for them to parent their grandchildren.

I care for a number of families where the grandchildren are cared for by their grandparents for a variety of circumstances: the death of a parent, a parent's chronic illness, and even the military deployment of a young mother. Each grandparent has eagerly and warmly welcomed these children into his or her life. The daily demands of caring for small children and their comforting routines have been a welcome diversion from their own grief, loss, and worry.

Despite these early challenges in their lives those children are fortunate to have their grandparents to step in when their parents were not able to care for them. All of the grandparents have intentionally helped even the youngest child to remember and honor their parents while clearly setting limits and maintaining the order their grandchildren need. I am in awe of how well most grandparents can rise to this challenge and find it a privilege to help care for their grandchildren.

Some families won't be fortunate enough to have grandparents in their lives, because of death or estrangement. In those cases, parents may choose to find an older friend to take on the role of grandparent in their children's lives. All children benefit from having the unconditional love of many people in their lives. Some adults without their own grandchildren will delight in having a small friend to dote on. Neighbors, members of faith-based organizations, distant relatives, and older family friends may all be touched to be asked to play such a special part in your child's life. We all love to feel needed and reaching out brings rich rewards.

Grandparents, near or far, play an exceptional role in their children's and grandchildren's lives. An added joy for grandparents is seeing their own children become parents. Grown children will treasure seeing their parents in a new light, as grandparents. My brothers and I remember going fishing with our grandfather. He would patiently bait our hooks and taught us all to cast safely. It has been a delight to see that scene replayed as our father goes fishing with my children, niece, and nephew.

When I was growing up we all knew the clear limits in our house; my mom had very clear expectations. I realized with a start that it was a new day when I saw her in her new role as grandmother. She was cheerfully encouraging my toddler daughter to dip French fries into her ice cream! It is a memory that to this day makes me laugh. Treasure your parents as grandparents and find ways to include them as valued members of your children's lives.

CHAPTER 22

Let's Go to the Park!

Keeping Children Active

Every neighborhood has its own fun places that a parent or child care provider can walk to with children, but I've found that children don't always need a special destination. They are happy to be outdoors in what feels to them to be a big, fresh, and new world. Just a walk around the block can be a big adventure and is both fun and healthful for children. Over the years they are always thrilled when I say, "Let's go to the park!"

I've been reading a lot lately that today's children don't get enough exercise. It's been reported that obesity is an increasing problem even among preschoolers. Maybe part of the problem is that kids don't walk enough or get outside to play.

We're lucky in Cambridge to have many neighborhood parks that are safe and within easy walking distance. Most of the children I've cared for over the years have been too young for organized sports, but they all loved to play in the park. Our local parks have playground areas suitable for little children as well as areas for the older kids. The tot areas have separate enclosures, with gates that can be securely shut to keep small children from running out into busy city streets.

In my old neighborhood the public library and a park were right across the street. The park was on spacious grounds that were part of the high school campus. In good weather I would take my child care group there, and they would run and kick a ball, play in the sandbox, or go down the slide. It was a good way for them to keep active before lunchtime and afternoon naps.

Of course, while a visit to any park is great fun for the kids, it requires constant vigilance on my part. Babies are easy to watch because they can nap safely tucked into a carriage or stroller, but it is amazing how quickly lively two year olds can get into mischief. They are forever tumbling and falling, crying for just a moment, but after a hug resuming play. There are always other children playing at the parks with their parents or child care providers, so the children from my group always find others to play with as well.

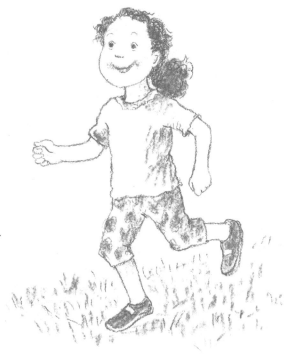

I've always tried to take advantage of what Harvard and the city of Cambridge have to offer for my child care groups. On the library grounds was a small amphitheater where I often took the children. They enjoyed watching a puppet show or short skit of a fairy tale, presented by the city's recreation department.

One of the many Harvard art museums was only a few blocks from my house, but it seemed like a real hike to the children. It had a lovely courtyard, with a goldfish pond. Museum staff enjoyed sitting at picnic tables during their lunch hour. During the summer, music from the museum's organ could be heard in the courtyard as well. On nice days we would join them during our lunchtime. Mesmerized by Bach and feeling very grownup to be sitting among the adults, the children were well behaved and were always most welcome.

Good behavior certainly was essential for attending local Harvard events such as the luncheon held under ancient elms on commencement day. It didn't matter that the children might forgo the chicken salad and rolls because they were always smiling when I took them over to the ice cream tent. With small paper plates on their laps, the children would sit

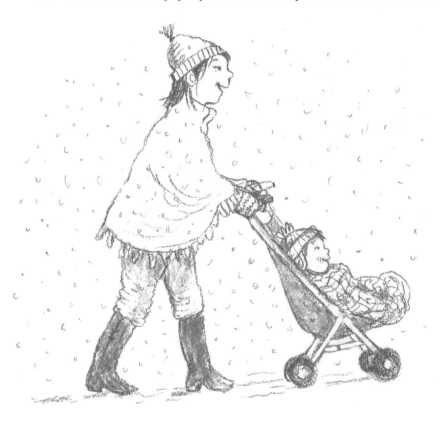

among the alumni and clap in delight, when the Harvard band marched past playing the college songs.

Walks to the parks and university grounds were both good exercise and a lesson in the rewards for good behavior. The children learned that I was only too pleased to take them for an outing when they held hands and followed directions.

Even during the winter months, on days when it wasn't too icy, we would take walks or go to the park to play in the snow. Sometimes on rainy days, the public library would happen to have a story hour. It was an opportunity for the children to learn to sit quietly while the librarian read them stories. In my current neighborhood, a popular nearby toy store also has a story hour, as does the local branch library.

Another exciting trip is a visit to the neighborhood firehouse. I've never met a firefighter who didn't enjoy showing the children the big hook and ladder fire engine. Sometimes they will even turn on the flashing lights and siren and give the kids firefighter hats and badges.

As Peggy has noted, children need active opportunities, frequently. A community initiative of the Cambridge Department of Public Health, *Healthy Living Cambridge*, attempts to encourage families to eat in a healthful fashion and stay active. The 5-2-1 campaign reminds us to eat five servings of fruit and vegetables a day, watch no more than two hours of television each day, and get at least one hour of physical exercise daily. These are useful guidelines for all families.

If you make exercise a part of your family's activities from the start, your children will grow up enjoying their active time and be better off for it. Start young, by taking those stroller babies out for walks on a daily basis. You and the baby will enjoy your outdoor time immensely. If you live in a northern climate and have to face winter, as we do, just bundle up the baby. My daughter was born in the cold snowy month of January, and it was a rare day that we didn't get outside for at least a short walk. My son was born in August, so we went for our walks in the evening when the weather had cooled off.

Toddlers love to go to the park. A grassy surface is the perfect surface on which to practice walking and, later, running. Many playgrounds now have areas with artificial surfaces that are quite forgiving when children fall. Time in a swing is a great thing for a toddler, too; think of how free they feel up in the air.

Preschoolers start to practice their gross motor skills at the park by climbing on playground equipment, sliding down the slides, and beginning to engage in games with other children. Meeting another parent and their children at the park is a nice way to socialize with other families. If you are new to an area, the local park is a great place to meet other families with young children.

Building in a little active playtime or exercise into your day when you are at home with your children is an easy thing to include and is often a high point of the day. For families who are juggling work and child care arrangements it takes a little forethought.

Depending on your commute to the child care center or caregiver's home, you may be able to walk there first with the stroller and then finish your commute to work on public transportation. That walk in the morning and on your way home in the evening can be your outdoor time together during the busy workweek. You will be amazed at what your child notices as the details of the neighborhood become familiar.

If you have to drive, keep a stroller in the car. On a beautiful spring morning you can leave the house a bit early and enjoy a nice walk with your child before you drop her off. Definitely build in some extra time because hurrying a young child anywhere isn't fun for either of you.

Another easy way to fit in some play time is to play with your child at a nearby park or the play area of the child care center after you pick him up and before you get into the car to leave. The child will be already dressed to go out and you won't be late, because it's the end of your day. The extra play time will be good for both of you, and you will arrive home ready for supper. If a child has had some active play with you at the end of the day, he or she may be a little better able to play independently while you fix the family meal.

The key is to make physical activity fun and simple and a regular part of your day.

To lead an active life you don't need an expensive gym membership or lots of exercise equipment—only the motivation to make it happen. On weekends, when you have more leisure time, plan a hike with the family, go bowling, or find a public pool that offers family swim time. Your children will be having so much fun they won't even realize that they are exercising.

When you do hire a child care provider or sign up at a center, make sure that they include plenty of opportunities for active play in the daily routine. Children can go out in most weather, at least for a short time, unless it's rainy or icy. Be sure you send your child with the right clothes and outer gear for the weather, including hats, mittens, and scarves to keep them warm and dry. An extra set of clothes, mittens, and socks are essential, especially in places where it gets cold and wet.

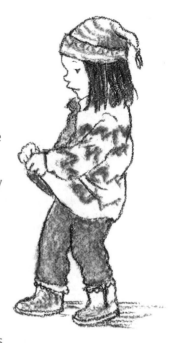

Because of their small size, children are more susceptible to extremes of temperature. When temperatures fall below freezing, and especially if there is significant wind, watch for early signs of overexposure to the cold. Frostnip is when exposed areas like fingers, cheeks, and the tip of the nose start to feel numb and look white. This is a sign it's time to go in and warm up. You can treat this at home by first removing any wet clothes, and then warming up the affected areas with gentle warm water (100 degrees Fahrenheit). There will be a tingling sensation as the affected area warms up.

Frostbite is much more severe and is a medical emergency. This is when affected areas are white, numb, and hard with actual freezing of the tissues. Once again, remove your child's wet clothes, wrap him in warm clothes and blankets, and bring him to a nearby hospital emergency room for rewarming therapy.

Extra water, a hat, and sunscreen are important when the children play outside in the summer. Remember to reapply sunscreen every two hours if your children are in the water. Try to avoid the intense times of peak sun exposure from 11 a.m. to 2 p.m. If the temperature rises into the high nineties or is very humid, children will need lots of breaks in the shade and plenty of water. If it is really hot, children may just want to sit in the shade of a big tree and listen to a story.

When you get to the stage your children can sometimes stay with a teenage baby-sitter, be sure to give the sitter ideas for safe and active play as well so the teen doesn't just park the children in front of the television while you're away. With a little prompting a sitter can take the children to the park, kick around a soccer ball with them, or help them fly a kite.

Children who spend more time playing outside and being active will be spending less time in front of a video, electronic game, or television screen. The correlation between more hours of screen time and a greater risk for obesity has been repeatedly confirmed. Seeing less television and watching fewer commercials for sugary beverages and high-calorie snack foods will have a positive influence on children's eating habits as well.

Some families live in neighborhoods where it is not safe to send the children outside to play. In that case, look around for alternative indoor locations to be active. Shopping malls provide great indoor walking space year-round, and some even have walking clubs and activity promotions. They are also easy places to take a baby in a stroller. Many high schools, colleges, and universities open their gyms, tracks, and pools to families when the athletes aren't practicing.

Even little changes in your behavior as a family can make the difference. When you run out of milk, take the time to walk together to the store instead of driving the short trip. When you do go to a mall, park far away and walk to the stores instead of circling for the closest parking space. In buildings where it is safe to take the stairs, walk down, and even think about walking up.

As adults, positive health habits we initiate at a young age are more likely to be consistently maintained than the ones we try to add when we are older. By nurturing your young children's love of physical activity, you will be helping them to stay healthy and active for the rest of their lives.

CHAPTER 23

Our Busy Lives

Scheduling and Overscheduling Children

Whatever became of those wonderful expanses of time, filled with hours of unsupervised play that children of my generation enjoyed? There seemed to be endless stretches of time for play, especially before we entered kindergarten at what now seems to be the advanced age of five. Most of the children I care for these days are off to nursery school or pre-school by the time they are three or four years old.

I'm pleased that some of the children continue to stay with me for a half day after their morning preschool and we can continue to enjoy each other's company. Many will come and join the others at lunchtime, take a much-needed nap, enjoy stories, and play in the afternoon. We have time to catch up and they tell me all about the many things they do at school and at home. Goodness, they do seem to have very busy lives.

I have cared for children as young as two when they began taking classes at the nearby Longy School of Music. Art, ballet, and swimming lessons are also popular enrichment activities for the local preschool set. When they are a little older they often join soccer teams and play Little League baseball, starting with the earliest level of tee ball.

These are all fun and healthy activities, which no doubt help children develop useful social skills and promote interaction with their peers. My only reservation about all these activities is that children never seem to have a moment to just relax and play. Some children may even seek a quiet moment alone, playing with favorite toys or looking through books. It seems to me that too often fun has to be organized.

In my day care, children always have time to participate in free play. In my view it is so important for children to have fun in an imaginative, unstructured way. When I was a little girl growing up in the 1930s I had lots of time to play with my sister Rose and the neighborhood kids. Hopscotch and jump rope were favorite summer games. In the winter, after a snowstorm, our brothers taught us how to "belly flop" down the path in the nearby park, using a trash barrel cover for a sled.

None of us ever went to day care or attended preschool; in fact, neither existed then. The neighborhood mothers would keep an eye on the kids whose mothers had to go off to work. We did hear that rich kids took piano and dance lessons, which would have been nice, but we didn't miss what we never had.

There was no Little League in those days or organized soccer teams. The neighborhood boys just played sports like baseball or basketball, coaching and supervising themselves. Until we went to kindergarten and were old enough to do household tasks, younger children were free to play freely as long as we behaved.

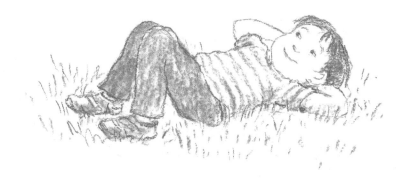

After we grew up both my sister Rose and I loved the book *A Tree Grows in Brooklyn* by Betty Smith and the movie later made from it. We could identify with Francie and her brother Neeley, who didn't have many material things as children but did have lots of fun.

Dick grew up as an only child. He says that back in the 1930s it never occurred to his parents that he was missing out on anything. Good manners, remaining quiet in the presence of grownups, and remembering to say bedtime prayers were their only expectations.

He was free to play in his backyard in Connecticut with neighborhood friends. He also has fond memories of Vermont summers spent with his grandparents. He often talks about spending lazy hot August afternoons lying in the grass behind his grandma's house, just watching clouds drift across the sky. In his daydreams those clouds soon became great white ships sailing to a faraway kingdom by the sea.

He selected a yellow canvas wigwam from the Sears and Roebuck catalog, and after it arrived he played Indian for much of the summer. His campsite was under the apple tree down by the barn, and he used currants from the garden as face paint for painting decorations on his face. He even wore a headdress of colored feathers purchased from the local "5 & 10" variety store.

Using a magnifying glass to reflect the sun, he learned to burn Mohawk symbols he discovered in a book into birch bark. Nowadays, he says, such activity might pass as precocious anthropological research, but he was only playing.

Dick has said that his seemingly passive, often solitary childhood did offer some benefits. Growing up, he discovered that daydreams are often a prelude to reality. He has rarely been lonely throughout his life and enjoys many activities he can do on his own: reading, listening to music, taking long walks, and jogging.

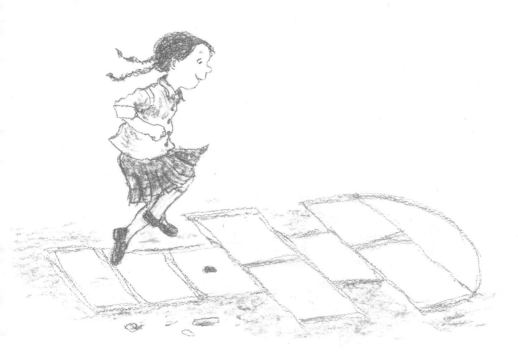

Children are social beings and truly enjoy the friends they make in day care and preschool. Our children had time to play with friends and also enjoyed playing alone in their rooms with favorite toys. Of course, they were young before preschool was in vogue and readily available. Both remember spending happy hours in the local park with me.

Every child is an individual—some enjoy always being in a crowd, while others appreciate quiet time alone to play, read, or just daydream. I encourage parents to listen and be attentive to their children and to try and include the types of activities or time for solitary play that they may need in their busy lives. All parents want the best for their children. I always suggest to parents that they try to include some quiet moments for them. We can't turn back the clock and give all children long lazy afternoons gazing at clouds, but we need to remember that children, like adults, need time to "just be."

Dick likes to quote the French essayist Montaigne: "The greatest thing in the world is to know how to belong to oneself." What a wonderful lesson that is to teach our children.

Peggy and Dick have wonderfully described some of the joys of a simpler time. As they have also noted, we can't turn back the clock. The lives of most families are quite different today. Parents and children live busier lives in a more complex fashion, but the key is to provide our children with some of the delights of an earlier, unstructured time.

The lives of families with young children are busy during the week with work, child care, and preschool schedules. Add in time to commute in the car or on public transportation and the time at home for supper, bath and story time, as well as homework squeezed in for older children, is very short.

I suggest that families make time to relax together on weekends and holidays. Parents can even use a precious vacation day during the summer to just have a relaxed day at home. A stretch of time playing at the park, when your children get to go home only when they are tired, is a true joy, as is a long sunny summer day at the beach. As Peggy noted with her own children, your children will remember those days fondly.

Growing up in the early 1960s, I too had hours of unstructured play. I remember hours sitting in a large tree in the neighbor's yard, with three other friends, acting out scenes from Johann David Wyss's novel *The Swiss Family Robinson*. We spent time riding our bicycles and playing pick-up baseball games in different backyards. Activities for children were just starting to be available, so I did take piano lessons, and practice, though probably not enough. My mother wisely wanted us all to learn to swim for safety and for fun, so my brothers and I took swimming lessons.

From an early age, children need to be encouraged to play independently. Even a very young baby from the age of four to six months can enjoy watching other children or batting the playthings on an activity gym structure on her own without a grownup interacting with her at the same time. Surround a toddler with a pile of blocks and let him be; the results will surprise you. Sometimes an older child of three or four who states emphatically, "I'm bored," may need a little encouragement to build something or imagine a story for tiny people or animals to act out. Helping your child enjoy imaginative play on his own is a rich experience and a gift that fosters enjoyment of solitary pastimes as well as activities with friends.

Children also need unstructured time in their lives to decompress from the daily routine if they are in a child care setting or participate in many activities. The best child care settings, regardless of type, include some time for unstructured play every day. Young children need time to relax and unwind just as their parents do. I have seen very young children with stress-related physical symptoms, such as headaches and stomach aches caused by pressure-filled, fast-paced lives. This can be avoided with careful attention to what kind of time and activities your child needs.

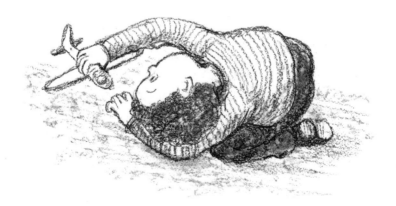

Taking a moment to sit together to read a story with your child when you come in the door at night is a pleasant way to reconnect after a day apart and the commute home. Children might need a light snack of some fruit or a carrot stick or two while you prepare supper. If you take the time to reconnect first, fixing the family meal may be a bit easier. What your children need most are your attention, time, and love. If you can meet their needs for these essential elements, the rest is much less critical.

Even in the midst of our busy lives, taking a moment to be with your child and appreciate life together is a joy to be treasured. Take a short walk down the block, enjoy your bus ride home together, or listen to a fun children's music tape in the car coming home from work and child care. Children love to notice a colorful sunset, a full moon, or a rarely seen rainbow. You will build rituals, treasured memories, and teach your child the joys of savoring life's little pleasures.

I encourage parents to jot down or record some of the many things their children say or do; they grow up quickly, and you will find that later it is hard to remember everything. As children grow, they will enjoy reading their book, listening to an audiotape, or watching a videotape and learning about their own accomplishments. They will love to hear exactly what they did say when they were two. Whether in the format of a baby book, scrapbook, or electronic journal, it will become a treasured keepsake.

With some thoughtful attention to the pace of their lives and yours, you can focus on what will be truly meaningful to your children. Both the rhythm and the content will make a big difference to you and your children at every stage.

CHAPTER 24

Transitions

Helping Young Children Cope with Change

Young children don't like change. They draw a sense of security from following a daily routine that allows them to predict what will happen next. I find they often want to find everything in the same place as it was yesterday in my home. I've also observed that children can be remarkably resilient when dealing with a small change such as a new preschool or a monumental change such as a parental divorce.

The first big transition most children have to cope with is leaving their parents and familiar surroundings to come and spend time with me or another caregiver. Most of the children in my care come to me when they are about two to three months old. It seems to be a good age to begin child care, and it's often when many mothers have to return to work outside the home. When babies are that young, it's easy for them to adapt to a different environment, especially one where other children are happily playing.

I advise new parents not to to tiptoe silently about the house when their baby is asleep. Infants quickly become accustomed to normal household sounds. Parents should consider that when their baby is cared for outside the home it is unlikely that she will be sleeping in a quiet room.

Parents can help prepare their babies for this early transition. I ask parents to write out their baby's feeding and sleeping schedule for me.

I also like to know whether it is necessary to follow it precisely. I have come to find that babies vary greatly in their needs. Some will eat and sleep on an almost precise timetable while others will fluctuate from day to day.

When I began taking care of Lila, she was almost three months old. Although her mother was nursing her, she began introducing a bottle well before Lila came to stay with me. With this preparation, I never had a problem getting Lila to take her bottle. She was one of those "clockwork" babies who wanted to be fed every three hours. You could set your watch by her.

With proper preparation, the baby's transition to day care from home can go smoothly. I find that the transition is often as much or more challenging for the mother than for the baby. I ask parents to pack a bag containing the following and bring it daily to my home:

» Transitional object (favorite stuffed toy or blanket).
» Diapers.
» Change of clothes.
» Telephone numbers: home, work, and mobile phone numbers for both parents.
» Emergency contact information to use in the event I can not reach a parent.
» Pediatrician contact information.
» Breast milk or formula for infants.

Right from the start I try to get the baby used to our routine, and most fit in quite well in a short time. With older children, I also emphasize our daily routine and follow a predictable schedule to help them make sense of their day and know what to expect. On a daily basis all children have to cope with their parents leaving. From the beginning of their time with me as infants, I encourage their parents to wave goodbye when they leave in the morning. When the children are older, they wave goodbye themselves to their parents from the window and enjoy that part of their morning as well.

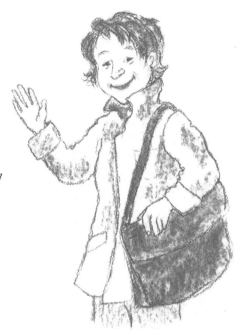

It helps a child to accept that mommy or daddy's coming and going is part of the daily routine.

In many years of providing child care, I haven't found separation anxiety to be too much of an issue, especially for children who start with me as babies. It may be a bit more difficult when children start with me at six to twelve months old, and also between eighteen and twenty-four months because it is normal for them to experience this anxiety at these ages. They are so much more aware then of the difference between their parents and other caregivers. I always suggest that parents leave quickly in the morning so the child can become comfortable with the other children and our daily routine. Within a couple of days the child will look forward to coming to my house and playing with new friends.

The next transition many children face is going off to preschool at age three or four or kindergarten at age five. When the children in my group go off to school, I'm excited for them but sad to see them leave; each child becomes an important part of my life.

Some of the children in my care leave to go to full-day preschool at age three. Some may start a part-time preschool where they go to school for anywhere from three to five hours a day several days a week and spend the rest of the day with me. Other children attend preschool two or three full days each week and spend the rest of the week with me. These are good options for parents whose schedules can accommodate them because it eases the transition for all of us and may meet the child's developmental needs better than going right to a full-day program. It also ensures that the child has some time for unstructured play and a nap during the day, which many children still need at ages three and four.

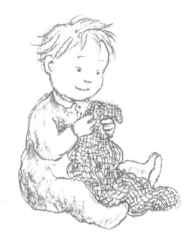

The older children who have gone off to full-time preschool or kindergarten, my "alums," still love to have a "Peggy Day" when they come back to join us. They may come on a day when school is closed for too much snow up here in the Northeast or on a minor holiday such as President's Day when many parents have to work. The younger children love having the older ones around as well.

I truly enjoy the days when the older children come back. It's a delight to see them and hear about all their adventures. I feel a little like the old schoolmaster in James Hilton's story *Goodbye, Mr. Chips*, when he recalls all the students whose lives he had touched and influenced in a positive way. Often my "alums" come back after they graduate from high school or college and even after they marry. I recently had the thrill of holding in my arms the lovely daughter of one of my "alums," now grown and married. I hope to have that baby in my child care group as well.

Another challenging transition for young children is moving. Children experience change on a personal level, so a move may seem unnecessary and scary. Our own daughter was very upset when we moved when she was two. She had a favorite rug covered with a pattern of pink, white, and blue teddy bears, which she hugged tightly after it was rolled up for the move. She was afraid we weren't going to take it with us. Of course we took it because we wanted her new room to look as much as possible like her old room. Both she and her stuffed animals quickly settled into the new place and, as it turned out, we didn't move again until the children were grown up.

I find that children do best with moving when they are properly prepared. They need to hear lots of stories of what it will be like when they arrive at where they are going. Even if they are going off somewhere far away, which is often the case in our bustling academic community of Cambridge, children need to be reminded that they will have friends wherever they go and that their parents will always care for them. I enjoy getting postcards and holiday greetings from families who have moved as far away as the Seychelles, Canada, South Africa, and Israel.

Although many transitions are happy ones and a positive part of growing up, sadly, some are not. Separation and divorce are major upheavals in the life of a child. Children may have to move and adjust to life with each parent in separate homes. As a child care provider, I have tried scrupulously not to take sides. I want what is best for each child, and I try to remain on good terms with both parents.

During a divorce or other significant changes in a child's life, I often observe some changes in the child's behavior. It may be helpful to the parents for me to comment on these behaviors. For example, a child in a very contentious divorce was often sad and tearful and required lots of hugs and holding. He was seeing less and less of one parent because of the circumstances. I was able to intervene and suggest some changes in parents alternating pick-up and drop-off times that helped the child feel more secure.

Fortunately, I haven't had much direct experience with a death in the families of the children in my care. There have been several occasions where a grandparent has died. Families handle death differently, depending on their cultural and religious traditions. One family was very straightforward with a young child, telling her that her grandfather had died and gone to heaven and that his presence was with them at the wake and funeral. Other families are much more indirect, mentioning the death only in whispers and preferring to let the child gradually sense the grandparent is no longer around.

When my sister Rose's husband died, her two little girls were two and five years old. My sister, understandably grief stricken, asked me to tell the girls that their Daddy wouldn't be coming home from the hospital, that he had gone to heaven. The older child said, "That's good; Daddy can get better in heaven and come home soon." Sadly, I had to explain that her daddy could only be better in heaven and wouldn't be coming home. We would all miss him, but he would wait for us in heaven. This seemed to be comforting to my niece, and she went back to playing with her dolls.

It's never easy to explain death, especially to a child. Parents will usually rely on the beliefs and traditions of their family and faith. Most children simply accept the explanation of the loss, and with their natural resilience eventually move on and accept this heart-wrenching transition.

Peggy is right: children are remarkably resilient. Whether coping with major emotional upheaval or the arrival of a new child in their child care setting, children will do well, especially if the adults pay close attention to what they need. For all transitions the basics are the same in supporting young children. Children need to know they are loved, that they will be well cared for by their parents, and that anything that has gone wrong is not their fault.

With the first transition from home to child care, it is important to give the new caregiver all the tools to help the baby succeed. This means teaching your breastfed baby to drink from a bottle or sippy cup in advance of starting child care.

Some breastfed babies absolutely refuse to take a bottle from their mothers but will readily accept it from anyone else. In a pinch, a recalcitrant baby new to day care can be fed with a cup or even a dropper until he or she takes good volumes of pumped breast milk or formula in a bottle. If your baby is four to six months old when starting day care and has been exclusively breastfed, he may be happiest going straight to a cup and skipping bottles.

Peggy has laid out the essentials nicely for helping a baby succeed in the transition to day care. Understanding a baby's preferences helps the caregiver feel successful and the baby feel more secure. Beloved objects help the baby feel at home, and sticking more or less to the same schedule helps the routine to feel familiar as well.

Her description of children waving goodbye brings back memories of my own children, when they were small, waving goodbye at that same window. Prior to finding Peggy, I had my own ups and downs with a variety of caregivers, including one that triggered an excruciating bout of separation anxiety in my daughter as a toddler.

Heading off to work with a screaming toddler clinging desperately to my leg was a terrible experience for both of us! That was the moment that I learned best to trust my own instincts: if I didn't feel comfortable leaving my child, it probably wasn't the right child care situation. My children settled in quickly at Peggy's and truly enjoyed their days with her. Dropping off the children and picking them up in the evening became wonderful bookends to my day.

With an upcoming transition to preschool, a new child care setting, or even kindergarten, children need to be prepared in advance. Although their concept of time may be fuzzy, give them time to adjust. Tell him, "After summer, you'll be going to a new school for kindergarten." Take advantage of any visiting days the new child care setting, preschool, or kindergarten offers. Walking by the school— and talking about what is inside and what their day will be like—helps children to start to imagine themselves in the new setting. Allowing children to say goodbye at the old school or child care is also very important in ensuring successful transitions.

Most of the time, the transition to preschool or kindergarten is determined by your child's chronological age and the cutoff dates established in your community. If your child has a birthday very close to the cutoff date, be sure that he or she is really ready. Sometimes extra time in a less-structured setting is just what a child needs to feel confident and secure before moving on.

Some children may be ready for a more challenging setting before the time they meet the age criteria. In that case, you may need to search for a more unusual option such as a prekindergarten class or a transitional year in a mixed-group classroom. If you have concerns about your child's readiness or placement, speak with your pediatrician. The school department in your town can be helpful as well in providing an evaluation of your child.

Moving can be a stressful transition for young children. Like most older children and adults, young children don't like change, especially at first. Many of the reasons that excite parents about moving, such as more space, a new job, or a different city are unimportant in the eyes of a young child.

Acknowledging their feelings and giving them a chance to express them will help them adjust to the inevitable move. Children do best with moves when their daily routine can be kept as consistent as possible. Try to set up the child's room as soon as possible for a nap on moving day and bedtime at the usual time.

Routines are very reassuring to a young child coping with the inevitable transitions that accompany a divorce. Remember to reassure your child that she is loved by both parents and will be well cared for and that whatever disagreements there may be between the parents, this is not her fault. It is useful for parents to come up with a very simple, developmentally appropriate explanation that they can stick to when answering questions, such as "Mommy and Daddy have had some grown-up problems that can't be fixed and make it impossible for us to all live together."

It is also important to tell your children the truth. It undermines their sense of safety and reality if they are told everything is fine, and they know it is not. Saying that the other parent will return to live with you, when you know they won't, is not helpful. It is best to gently and firmly let your child know that, difficult as it is, their parents will not be living together again. This helps the child adjust to the new reality and move on. Being prompt for pick-up and drop-off time builds goodwill between parents and is reassuring to the child. Sticking to these routines and keeping the conflict out of sight of the child are the two most constructive things divorcing parents can do for their children.

Routines that are stable and predictable help both parents and children cope with the many transitions of divorce.

Building in special routines at transition times, such as always waving goodbye at a certain place or reading a special "hello" story together after the child is dropped off after a stay at the other parent's house, can be very helpful.

Sometimes in divorce, because of substance abuse, domestic violence, child abuse and neglect, or other critical circumstances, one parent is unable to function in his or her role. In this case it is imperative that you, as the only parent available to your child, are very consistent and clear in your behavior and expectations.

Reassure your child often that she will be safe and well cared for. When one parent is not present for a long period of time, explain this very simply to your child. "Mommy can't take care of you, because she has been very sick, and has to go away for a long time and get better."

If a child has witnessed violent behavior, it is very important to let her know that she will be safe. "Daddy couldn't control his temper and be safe, so now he has to go away for a long time and get help to learn how to be safe." As children grow, they return to the difficult situations in their past and will ask more detailed questions at each developmental stage.

The remaining parent in a difficult transition also carries the double burden of coping with his or her own feelings of loss, anger, and fear as well as supporting the child. This is a time when outside therapeutic support is indicated to shore up your own emotional resources and help you be the parent you want to be for your child. Children are gifts to their parents during divorce and other challenging transitions, because they keep the adults focused in the present and ready for the ever-present demands of parenting.

The death of a parent is a life-altering transition for young children. Children who have lost a parent need to have ample opportunity to grieve in an age-appropriate fashion. Children will continue to return to that loss at different developmental stages to reexplore their feelings. The impact is very much affected by the child's developmental stage and by the other people and supports surrounding the child at the time of the loss. Support groups for children who have lost a parent are invaluable in these circumstances.

Dealing with a death in the family and parenting a young child at the same time is a particular challenge for the surviving adult as well as the child. The adult must deal with his or her own grief and loss and still care for and support the child. Professional support in the form of individual or group therapy is essential in this situation for adults as well.

Young children do not respond to loss and death in the same way as adults. They may be very matter of fact and almost disinterested. Death will not seem final to them. They will keep asking whether the person will come back and then return to playing cheerfully. For everyone's sake, settle on a very simple explanation and stick to it. "Grandpa's body was old, tired, and sick, and it just stopped working. It can't be fixed." Brace yourself for endless questions about why and whether he is just sleeping.

Transitions, change, and loss are all inevitable parts of life. As you face these transitions together, remember to prepare your child in advance if possible. Remind her she is loved and well cared for. You will be setting a powerful example for your children as you show them how to survive and embrace change, live through loss, and continue to celebrate with joy the positive transitions in life.

Afterword

Just One More Thing

Relax. As new parents you'll undoubtedly do the right thing in caring for your baby. All parents have an instinctive gift for nurturing their newborns and will want to protect and provide the best of everything for their child.

My brother-in-law drove us home from the hospital with our firstborn, our daughter Wendy. Harry asked whether I was nervous. "No," I laughed, "I'm excited and happy, but not nervous. After all, I'm not the first woman to have a baby!" It's true: for the most part you'll just do what comes naturally.

Wendy was born in July. One night shortly after we took her home to our Cambridge apartment there was a wild, "crash bang" midsummer thunderstorm. At the sound of a big thunderclap both Dick and I leaped from our bed to check on Wendy, certain she would be terrified by the noise. We found her sleeping peacefully in her crib and the noise of the storm could just as well have been a lullaby. We laughed at ourselves, and the fear we shared for our baby girl, but it was perfectly normal for us to be concerned. We reacted instinctively, just as every good parent does.

Dr. Lisa and I hope that our little book has been fun to read and practical and that the stories we've shared from our years of experience will be helpful in raising your young children. Nevertheless, as parents, be assured that your instincts will assist you in many different child care situations. Also, common sense will help you know when to seek medical care for your baby.

It's no surprise how ideas and opinions seem to come full circle. More mothers are now breastfeeding, which was frowned upon as being old-fashioned when my children were born. Years ago, families grew their own food and ate fresh produce from their farms and gardens. Young families today seem to be paying much more attention to what their children eat and organic foods are becoming much more widely available.

We see these changes and more in our own family. With our grand-children Teddy and Pru, their mother Jane made all their baby food in a blender from fresh organic fruit and vegetables. They thrived on breast milk and fresh produce much as though they had been born in an earlier

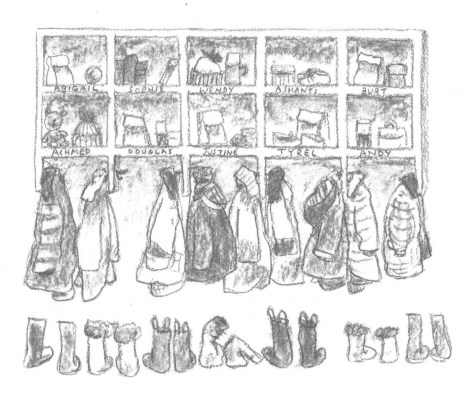

century. Teddy and Pru have had the best of what is natural and at the same time the benefits of modern medicine, preventative care, and immunizations. They have the best of both worlds. Teddy is a sturdy little fellow who loves to run about in his parents' English garden, and his sister Pru toddles close behind.

You might say that, in the long run, your children will probably be very much like yourselves. Almost all of the children I've cared for over the years I would consider to be privileged, and not necessarily in a monetary sense. Most important of all, they have been fortunate in having loving and caring parents. Unless they make poor choices, these children have been given every chance to live happy productive lives.

In several of the stories I have shared I've mentioned that I came from a large, less privileged, and motherless family. In retrospect it's clear that, at times, we really were poor, but we always loved and cared for each other. My siblings and I all look back fondly at the many good times we shared and laugh at the tougher times. I have always considered my own immediate family to be both privileged and fortunate. The *most* important gifts parents can give their children are *your* love and attention. We hope you have enjoyed our book.

Trust your instincts, and follow your heart as a parent.

In the end, I agree once again with Peggy. For those of us blessed with good role models in our own families we are fortunate to have a clear path to follow. For those who seek to raise their children differently, perhaps in a different part of the country, or even a different culture, it is useful to have some clear direction. For all parents, we hope our book will encourage you to become a more thoughtful parent, answer some of your questions along the way, and help you enjoy your children as they grow.

A charming children's book, *Bub; or, The Very Best Thing* by Natalie Babbitt, says in such a tender way that love *is* the best gift you can give your children. Knowing that they are the center of your world helps them grow into sturdy, competent children. Sometimes the days with small children can seem endless, with all the fuss, mess, meals, and cleanup. In the scheme of a lifetime, these moments with small children are fleeting. Make the most of them, enjoy them, and treasure them as much as possible. We hope we have given you the tools to make your journey as parents intentional, enjoyable, and memorable.

WEB-BASED AND OTHER RESOURCES FOR PARENTS

---

www.aap.org

American Academy of Pediatrics. Comprehensive information for parents and professionals on children's health issues and advocacy.

www.naeyc.org

National Association for the Education of Young Children, an organization for educators and families. Useful information about choosing an accredited preschool.

www.kidshealth.com

Nemours Foundation's Center for Children's Health Media. Engaging and accurate health information written at different levels for children, teens, and parents.

www.cdc.gov

Centers for Disease Control. Up-to-the-minute information about health issues around the world. Particularly useful for parents traveling overseas with children.

www.cbcbooks.org

Children's Book Council, an organization of children's book publishers. Includes a very nice reading list *Books to Grow On* for children, from newborns to three year olds, chosen by the American Library Association and the Children's Book Council Joint Committee.

www.ror.org

Reach Out and Read, a Boston-based pediatric literacy organization. Provides information for parents about reading to their children and information for pediatricians and other health care providers to become involved in promoting literacy.

www.rif.org

Reading Is Fundamental (RIF), the venerable nonprofit literacy organization. Identifies activities for kids and reports interviews with children's authors and information about starting a program.

www.ala.org/aslc/awardsscholarships

Association for Library Service to Children, a division of the American Library Association. Complete information about the Newberry and Caldecott Medals and other awards, as well as lists of all winners. Also includes a wealth of information about children's literature and authors.

INDEX

numbers for, 61; planning for, 139. *See also* Safety issues

Encouragement for parents, 194–97

EpiPen®, 64

Erikson, Erik, 75

Exercise, 168–75

Expectations of children, 9–11, 13–16

Families, 33–39; blended, 34, 108–9; bringing second child into, 7, 104–6; moving of, 187, 190–91; traditions of, 36; transitions in, 7–8, 183–93; variations of, 33–34

Family stories, 162–64

Fast foods, 58

Fathers, 1–3, 6–7

Feeding baby. *See* Eating/feeding

Fever, 19, 24–25; treatment of, 25–26

Finger foods, 56

Firehouse visits, 171

Flexibility: to change plans, 14–15; of child care schedule, 18

Flexible benefits plans, 25

Food allergies or sensitivities, 52, 60–64

Front packs for babies, 75–76

Frostbite, 174

Gay parents, 38–39

Gifts: for care provider, 26; for good behavior, 111–12, 152

Good manners/behavior, 110–17, 170; discussions about, 116; expectations for, 117; modeling, 111, 113, 117; praise for, 111–13; teaching, 113–14, 117; while traveling, 129, 131

Grandparents, 7–8, 37, 161–67; as child's caretakers, 4, 161, 166–67

Halloween, 20

Hay fever, 61

Health kit for travel, 134–35

Hearing screening, 27

Heat exposure, 174

Hitting, 94–100

Holidays, 20, 35

Honesty, 114–15, 191, 192

Household tasks, 14–15, 115–16

Ibuprofen, 25

Imagination: fear and, 138; in play, 145–52

Infections: ear, 29; transmitted by pets, 125

International adoption, 34, 42–43, 45

International travel, 134

Internet resources, 199–200

Introducing solid foods, 55–56, 62–63

Juices, 56–57, 58

Kicking, 96–99

Kindergarten, 185–86, 190

Kosher diet, 52

Latchkey kids, 10

"Lazy" eye, 28–29, 30

Lesbian parents, 38–39

Library visits, 154–55, 158, 168, 171

Limit setting, 9–17

Love, 197

Lunch. *See* Eating/feeding